THE AWARD-WINNING VIDEO

"Sawyer Mac has hit all the right notes here . . . Appropriate definitions, excellent information, clear demonstrations, and [graphical] inserts keep the information easy to understand and follow. . . . This tape would be valuable in all public libraries and pediatricians' offices."

—*Library Journal*

"In what may possibly be the greatest head lice movie ever made . . . HEAD LICE TO DEAD LICE is a funny, but delicately handled, look at a potentially embarrassing but common health problem. Highly Recommended."

—*Video Librarian*

"Frantic parents and their itching offspring now have recourse in a five-step 'battle plan' outlined in a humorous, disarming and easy-to-follow award-winning fifteen-minute video, HEAD LICE TO DEAD LICE."

—*Health Digest*

"An unceasingly spreading public health problem is given close examination, explanation, and therapeutic recommendation in a manner which children and adults will appreciate for its knowledgeable treatment and witty presentation . . . This comic video offers the remarkable opportunity to laugh about a condition countless families have experienced."

—*Children's Video Review Newsletter*

"I commend your efforts to identify treatments for head lice that are effective, safe, and provide an alternative to traditional methods. . . . Your video, HEAD LICE TO DEAD LICE was informative and amusing."

—Richard J. Pollack, Ph.D., entomologist,
Harvard School of Public Health

"Admiration for a job extremely well done must be expressed . . . Not only is it highly instructive but also entertaining. Wish we could have used it when I was teaching about lice at CDC. Timing is excellent as the head-louse epidemic continues to expand across the world."

—Harold George Scott, Ph.D.,
world famous entomologist and lice expert

"This video tackles lice in a sensitive, humorous style . . . sure to relax the most squeamish parent."

—Kevin T. Kalikow, M.D., Asst. Clinical Prof. of
Child Psychiatry, New York Medical College

HEAD LICE TO DEAD LICE

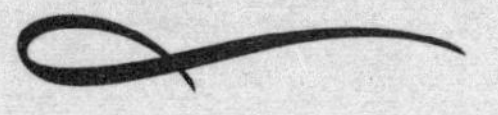

Joan Sawyer
&
Roberta MacPhee

St. Martin's Paperbacks

HEAD LICE TO DEAD LICE

ISBN: 0-312-97260-1

Printed in the United States of America

St. Martin's Paperbacks edition/ November 1999

St. Martin's Paperbacks are published by St. Martin's Press, 175 Fifth Avenue, New York, N.Y. 10010.

10 9 8 7 6 5 4 3 2 1

AUTHORS' NOTE

This book is for informational purposes only and is not intended to take the place of advice from a trained medical professional.

The authors would like to thank . . .

. . . **Mary Ward,** who has always made herself available to us and to everyone else who has needed help in conquering head lice.

. . . **Harold George Scott,** Board-Certified Entomologist, for writing the preface and for generously going through this entire manuscript with the proverbial fine-tooth comb, correcting not only every scientific inaccuracy but also every comma and period. And he did it in record time.

. . . **Dr. Richard Pollack,** Entomologist at the Harvard School of Public Health, who has always taken time from his busy schedule to answer our questions patiently and to help so many head lice sufferers to identify their nits, lice, and dandruff.

. . . **Ilene Ungerleiter,** school nurse at the Cambridge Friends School, who has identified lice cases for us, tested numerous combs, and first gave us the chance and the encouragement to test the olive oil protocol.

. . . to our editor at St. Martin's Press, **Barry Neville,** who found us on the Internet and asked us to write this book.

. . . to our families—**Neil Shifrin, Lily Shifrin, Timothy Sawyer, Erica Sawyer, and Talia Sawyer**—for putting up with our long working hours.

And finally, a great big thank-you to the "young person" in our office, **Christine Manolis,** who kept our office running smoothly, kept us running smoothly, and even drew the pictures for this book.

We couldn't have done it without you!

Contents

How to Use This Book

What to do immediately if you find head lice on you or your child:

If you have found head lice on your child or yourself, don't panic. The program outlined in this book will help you deal with the problem. And don't worry about all the horror stories you've heard. Most of the problems associated with head lice are caused by incomplete or inaccurate information.

Yes, many head louse populations appear to have become resistant to available pediculicides. However, by following the Five-Step Battle Plan described in Chapter 4, you will be able to eliminate even the most chronic infestation. The Five-Step Battle Plan uses olive oil as a smothering agent to eliminate head lice and help remove the nits (lice eggs). You can read more about how and why olive oil works in Chapter 3.

First make sure you have the following items on hand:

Shopping List

- A great big bottle of the least expensive *olive oil* you can find. It doesn't have to be virgin or cold pressed. Pumice grade (olive oil in its crudest form) is usually best, if you can find it. This form is the least refined and contains more of the actual plant, which has many beneficial properties. Your local restaurant might sell you or your school a large can.

- A small plastic *applicator bottle* similar to the one used for applying color to hair.
- An over-the-counter pediculicide (if you choose to use one). Check with your physician or pharmacist for the one best suited for each member of your family. Remember, do not use anything containing Lindane (Kwell).
- Plastic shower caps.
- Bandannas.
- A good *metal nit comb* (see discussion of various nit combs on page 99).
- *Vision visor:* if you are visually challenged, you may want to consider getting one of these binocular magnifiers. They magnify two and a half times at 8 inches, and help you see the nits while leaving your hands free to pick nits. They look like goggles and you can wear them with or without glasses. We find that wearing this gives us confidence in determining what we're seeing, especially since we are over forty. To order call 1-888-DIE LICE.
- A good clarifying shampoo like Clairol Herbal Essence for Oily Hair or Prell.

- Clean white towels.
- Covered elastic hair bands or hair clips.
- Regular clean combs.

Always keep the listed items on hand. If you are prepared for a head-louse infestation, you will be much less likely to panic when you find evidence of lice on your child's head.

Next, turn to page 89 and complete steps 1 and 2 of the Five Step Battle Plan.

Once the olive oil is on everyone's head, grab a cup of tea, think how gorgeous your family's hair will look after this well-known beauty treatment, sit down, put your feet up, and finish reading Chapter 4, which outlines our Five-Step Battle Plan. Then read Chapter 3 for basic housecleaning tips.

And please, don't worry about head lice invading your house. These insects cannot live off a human scalp for more than thirty-six hours. While you will need to do some light housecleaning, the important work will be done on the human heads where head lice live, feed, and lay their eggs. After you have completed steps 1 and 2, you have time to sit down, read this book, and get ready to do battle.

Preface

Lice and their nits (eggs) have infested human heads since long before the beginnings of recorded history. Through eons of time they have been out of control, and they plague us still, as many temperate areas of Earth undergo head-louse epidemics.

Modern regimens have been developed that can eliminate and to some extent prevent head-louse infestations on individuals and within social groupings. Military units minimize the head-louse problem by requiring heads to be shaved or hair to be no longer than one-half inch.

With the development of laboratory-created pesticides just before and during World War II, scientists generated a long series of synthetic organic insecticides, some of which were superior louse killers. While many were so toxic to humans that their use could not be justified, others were widely and successfully employed over long periods of time. However, the specter of resistance emerged, causing these insecticides—one by one—to become less and less effective.

Resistance is a reflection of populations undergoing selection to produce survival of the fittest.

- Members of louse populations are individually variable.
- Individuals best suited for prevalent conditions have the greatest chance of surviving and reproducing.
- New generations will consist primarily of descendants of well-suited parents.
- An insecticide modifies conditions under which a louse must survive.
- Lice able to withstand the insecticide will survive to rebuild the population.
- Subsequent populations will exhibit ever greater resistance to that insecticide.

Resistance does not occur all at once. It develops over time in louse populations, so, in any particular location, both resistant and nonresistant populations may exist. This can cause much confusion because pediculicides [insecticides used to treat head lice] that work one day fail to work the next.

Authors Sawyer and MacPhee present an additional modern solution for head-louse infestations—use of olive oil—which bypasses the problems of toxicity and resistance. It is an extension of the concept presented in their videotape *Head Lice to Dead Lice*, which received the American Medical Association's Freddie Award in 1997 as best community health video in its International Film and Video Competition.

Of equal importance, the authors face up to

the problem of social stigma caused by louse infestation, recognizing that reduction of the current head-louse epidemic is not likely to occur unless and until lice come to be regarded as no more of a stigma than the common cold, until the public becomes thoroughly familiar with safe and effective approaches to control this ubiquitous creature.

Harold George Scott, Ph.D.
Board-Certified Entomologist

Letter from the Lice Ladies

Dear Fellow Parent:

Let me guess. You've just picked up your child, who has been sent home from school with—yuck!—head lice, or you have just heard another horror story from one of your friends about the nightmare of trying to get rid of those nasty little critters. You have vowed that if these pests even think about invading your nest, you're going to go after them with both barrels loaded.

Good for you!

Now, take a deep breath and get rid of all your old notions about who gets head lice. Because the truth is, everyone can get them. Trust us. We know. We talk to people who have them everyday. We talk to physicians, nurses, lawyers, teachers, everyone. These tenacious little insects have invaded the finest, most expensive private schools in the country. So, welcome to the dark side of parenthood. You're in good company.

Now, here's the good news. Head lice will not hurt your child permanently. There is no evidence that head lice transmit any diseases.

They are, however, somewhat tricky to get rid of.

Let us tell you a little story about the Sawyer family's experience with head lice, which inspired two middle-age moms to produce our award-winning video *Head Lice to Dead Lice: Safe Solutions for Frantic Families* and write this book.

Day 1

My good friend Lisa called to tell me that her kids had head lice and that since her kids had been playing with my kids, I should check my kids' heads carefully. She described the chemicals she had washed every head in the family with, the hours of cleaning and the backbreaking hours she had spent picking nits (louse eggs) out of her kids' heads. And she still couldn't get rid of the lice. In hushed tones, she whispered that she thought she was either losing her mind or that she was dealing with some kind of "mutant bug."

After I hung up the phone, I was less worried about head lice than I was about Lisa's mental health. She sounded to me like she was going 'round the bend. Immediately I thought of what a hard time she'd had lately. One of her closest friends had recently passed away from breast cancer. I thought she must have somehow associated head lice invading her children's heads with the invasive cancer that had taken her friend from her. Surely Lisa was overreacting.

I did what Lisa suggested and checked my kids. Of course, I had no idea what I was looking for, but Lisa had described the tiny creatures, the size of a sesame seed, and the hard-to-remove eggs. I found nothing that fit her description and decided my kids were fine. Just to make sure, I alerted their summer camp to check, in case I had missed something. The nurse called back and said all was well. I breathed a sigh of self-satisfied relief and forgot about it.

Day 7

My six-year-old daughter came down to where I was dutifully exercising my middle-age body with a Richard Simmons tape and complained that her head itched. Remembering Lisa's dire words of warning, I grabbed a flashlight and shone it on the spot Talia pointed out. There it was! A *louse!!* I grabbed it with my fingernails and ran shrieking upstairs to where my poor unsuspecting husband lay sound asleep in bed. It was, after all, 6:00 A.M. on Sunday morning.

I shook him none too gently and demanded that he wake instantly and take a look at what I had just pulled off my immaculately clean, healthy child. He struggled to comply with my near-hysterical demands. When his eyes were peeled open sufficiently, we put the specimen onto the bathroom counter to get a closer look. He did his guy thing and scrutinized it for a while, asking ridiculous questions like "How do you know it's a louse?" while in my mind I was already planning my assault on our heads and on our house to eliminate every single crawling creature that dared to invade my nest.

I flew into action, leaving him to poke at the louse. First, I found the yellow pages and located the closest all-night pharmacy. Armed with my trusty credit card, I tore out the door and went about implementing my usual problem-solving style—if you have a problem, throw money at it.

I bought plenty of Nix, metal nit combs, new brushes, regular combs, hair clips, rubber bands, and laundry detergent and went home, prepared to do battle. I read the directions on the Nix package carefully, fully aware that I was about to pour poison on my precious children's heads. Please understand that for the nine months I carried them in my womb, I had abstained from coffee, alcohol, and sugar to the point that my husband had to find a macrobiotic birthday cake for me. But now there were dastardly lice sucking the life's blood from my babies' scalps. I was going to destroy them and take no prisoners.

That day we Nixed, combed, picked, and cleaned. It took all day and was exhausting, but I ended up feeling virtuous and victorious. Surely I was a good mother. There was no sacrifice I was not willing to make for my children.

I kept my kids home from the last few days at camp, in case someone else had gotten lice and wasn't being as meticulous as I was. And I called in a visiting nurse to check my "picking" job. I left no stone unturned, Lisa's words of defeat echoing in my brain.

When I called Lisa and told her that we had, in fact, gotten head lice but now had things under control, she started to cry and had to hang up the phone. Oh, poor Lisa, get a grip, I thought. They're only insects.

Day 10

We left for vacation on Cape Cod armed with enough Nix for our second treatment. There we Nixed again on schedule, just to make sure.

Day 24

Upon our return from two weeks on Cape Cod, a professional nit-picker, (Mary Ward) who had extensive denitting experience in day care centers, came over for a professional recheck. Mary checked us in the backyard before any of us set foot in the house. But I was confident we had done everything right, and would therefore receive an A in head lice.

It didn't take Mary long to find new nits.

Okay, I thought, Lisa's words now eating their way through my stomach, here we go again. This time I went to the drug store and bought Rid (with a different active ingredient, pyrethrin instead of permethrin). And we started over, applying pesticide to my kids' heads now for the third time. Again we spent another precious day shampooing, combing, picking and cleaning. This time I called the Nix hotline. "What's going on?" I asked, none too kindly. "You advertise that this stuff works the first time."

"You must have gotten reinfested," she replied. "You must not have cleaned your house properly."

"We moved out of the house," I replied.

"Well, did you remember to change your vacuum cleaner bag?"

Oh, jeez, I thought. This is starting to feel like *The Twilight Zone.* Careful, I thought, you're starting to sound like Lisa. This time we went through the whole procedure under Mary's careful supervision.

She knew a lady close to a breakdown when she saw one, and, God bless her, she didn't leave my side until both kids were tucked, exhausted, into bed.

Day 29

We left for a scheduled, much-anticipated trip to England, again armed with pediculicides.

Day 31

There, in our London hotel room, we shampooed seven days later as directed on the package and used a product called Clear to "loosen the nits." I carefully hid the packaging in the garbage so the hotel staff wouldn't know we had head lice and throw us out into the street. Images of beggars living on the streets of London from the *Three Penny Opera* flashed into my poor jet-lagged brain. I kept telling myself I was overreacting. This time, surely, we were finished. We had now treated four times with chemicals. Just to be sure, I dragged a huge suitcase full of our clothes through the streets of London to a Laundromat and dried them in the hot cycle. One pair of expensive American Girl pajamas actually melted. Those English Laundromats do not mess around.

Day 33

We left London for a week in the Cotswolds. This village was so adorable, I expected to see Jemima Puddleduck, apron and all, around every corner. The cottage we rented was straight out of Beatrix Potter.

Day 38

As we hiked merrily to one of the ancient sites of mystically arranged stones, Talia's hand went up to scratch her head and my stomach clutched. I steeled myself and took a look. There it was. A louse!

We found a drugstore in one of the tiny villages and, while my family waited outside (they were more humiliated by my growing hysteria than by the lice), I marched inside. I waited to catch the eye of the young male chemist. Silently I beckoned with my finger, indicating my need for complete confidentiality. He came over; I'm sure expecting a confession of middle-age gonorrhea or something. When I asked what he had for head lice, he gave me a look and handed me a bottle. It contained malathion. I'd heard of malathion and it sounded harsh, but I was ready for harsh. Hell, I was ready to cut our heads off. He went on to assure me that it was no big deal. Many times the whole village treated themselves on the same day in order to deal with an epidemic.

I read the directions. They called for us to leave the malathion on our heads for twelve hours. Forget using this stuff in this adorable cottage with the 100-year-old paper-thin towels and dribbling makeshift shower.

That night we went home and picked in the dim light of a 200-year-old English country cottage. The next morning I had us booked in the most expensive hotel I could find in Bath. This was it, war! I needed thick towels and a major shower with some serious water pressure. The word "defeat" was not yet in my vocabulary.

Day 39

We checked into our expensive resort hotel, terrified our secret would be found out. Everyone else there was beautiful, thin, and (probably) lice-free. I felt old, ugly, fat, and infested. That night I carefully applied the poison to both of my daughters, my husband, then myself. We wrapped towels around our heads, and I promptly managed to lock myself out in the hallway in my caftan and turbaned head, trying desperately to make myself invisible as the beautiful people passed though the halls. Never in my life have I felt worse.

The next morning we took long, leisurely showers and checked out, $600 poorer. For the rest of our trip, we combed incessantly with our metal nit combs until our hair was so ripped up, we were unrecognizable.

Day 44

We continued to check our heads and found no more nits or lice.

When we got home I called my pediatrician and confessed what we had been through. When I mentioned the malathion he shrieked, "What! Haven't you read about kids getting malathion poisoning? Better you should have head lice!"

From there I spun into a vortex of guilt. What should I have done? How far should a good mother go to get rid of crawling creatures on her kids' heads? What should I have done differently? What was going on out there, anyway? If the stuff wasn't working, why wasn't anyone telling us?!!

I e-mailed my cousin in Israel, the entomologist, the father of two small children. "Do you get head lice in Israel?" I asked. "What do you do?"

"Oh, yes," he replied, "but I would never put pesticides on my kids' heads," thereby spinning my mother's guilt into new realms of agony.

"Okay, so what do you do?"

"We use olive oil," he replied, and went on to explain the procedure. Sure, it sounded messy, but a whole heck of a lot less guilt inducing. And messy I could deal with. Hadn't I changed some truly extraordinary diapers in my day? Hadn't I cleaned up not only my kids' but also their friends' carsickness? Compared to a carsick child, olive oil is *nothing*!

A few weeks later I received the dreaded notice in my child's lunch box. Head lice had invaded her classroom. Half the class and two of the three teachers had them. The only teacher spared was the man. Wouldn't you know it!

I grabbed my notes from my conversations with Moshe, my entomologist cousin, and headed for the school nurse. Fortunately, my kids go to a Quaker school in Cambridge, Massachusetts. This is about as liberal as you can get. They are not terribly uptight about head lice there. The school nurse checks heads right in the classroom, and they do math projects based on . . . "If you have four lice on your head and they each lay six eggs a day . . ."

Anyway, I told Ilene about the olive oil and she was intrigued. "Write it up," she suggested. "It can't hurt." Later that week we had half the parents willing to go along with the olive oil and half the parents convinced I was out of my mind. Since the package said Nix worked with one treatment, that's the route they were going. No old wives' tales for them! I was a hysterical mom and my kid didn't even have head lice this time.

Two weeks later all the kids who had used the olive oil were in school while the parents of the others, the ones who knew better, came to school to pick up their children and start the process all over again. They had "resprouted."

By the next week we had everyone using the olive oil—even the kids who didn't have head lice. They liked the way the other kids' hair looked. A few weeks later we had conquered the lice completely. Now I was getting phone calls from pediatricians who had gotten their hands on the information I had typed and wanted to know more. Parents had passed out the information in other schools where they had younger or older siblings.

The next time my writing group met, I told my saga of head lice. I turned to Roberta MacPhee, a fellow writer/film producer, mother, and all-around game person. "Hey," I said, "you wanna make a movie?" Thus was born Sawyer Mac Productions and *Head Lice to Dead Lice: Safe Solutions for Frantic Families*," and the story of two moms trying to spread the word about how to get rid of head lice without poisoning their kids.

So, here's what we've learned over the past two years. We hope that by reading this book and sharing our experience, you won't have to go through the frustration of battling a head louse infestation armed with outdated information.

Good luck and best wishes,

Joan Sawyer and
Roberta MacPhee
The Lice Ladies

Knowledge Is Power

1 Know Thy Enemy: Head Lice Through the Ages

Lice, or "cooties," as they have affectionately been dubbed, have been with humankind as long as people have been capable of scratching. Cave people were crawling with the little creatures, and scientists have found lice on the scalps of ancient Egyptian mummies. Why, even Cleopatra, Queen of the Nile, had her own solid gold nit comb. Rumor has it that Queen Elizabeth's elaborate white neck ruffle was worn to protect her clothing from lice. And haven't you ever wondered about those elaborate headdresses that covered the heads of women in medieval and Elizabethan times? In Williamsburg, Virginia, we learned that men wore wigs partly to protect themselves from head lice but since some wigs were made from infested human hair, it didn't always help.

The great Scottish poet Robert Burns was so impressed with one special louse that had the

Dead head lice have been removed from prehistoric mummies.

Lice are sometimes called cooties.

audacity to stroll along the bonnet of a fine lady that he immortalized it in his poem entitled:

To a Louse
On Seeing One on a Lady's Bonnet at Church
By
Robert Burns

Ha! whare ye gaun' ye crowlin ferlie?
[crawling marvel]
Your impudence protects you sairly;
I canna say but ye strunt rarely
Owre gauze and lace,

Tho faith! I fear ye dine but sparely
On sic a place.

Ye ugly, creepin, blastit wonner,
Detested, shunn'd by saunt an sinner,
How daur ye set your fit [feet] upon
her—
Sae fine a lady!

Gae somewhere else and seek your dinner
On some poor body.

Swith! [off!] in some beggar's hauffet squattle [temples squat];
There ye may creep, and sprawl, and sprattle [scramble];
Wi' ither kindred, jumping cattle;
In shoals and nations;

Whare horn nor bane ne'er daur unsettle
Your thick plantations.

Now haud you there! ye're out o' sight,
Below the fatt'rils [folderols], snug an tight,
Na, faith ye yet! ye'll no be right,
Till ye've got on it—

The vera tapmost, tow'rin height
O' Miss's bonnet.

My sooth! right bauld ye set your nose out,
As plump an grey as onie grozet [gooseberry]:
O for some rank, mercurial rozet [resin],
Or fell, red smeddum [deadly powder],

I'd gie you sic a hearty dose o't,
Wad dress your droddum [backside]!

I wad na been surpris'd to spy
You on an auld wife's flainen toy
[flannel cap]
Or aiblins [perhaps] some bit duddie
[small] boy,
On's wyliecoat;

But Miss's fine Lunardi [balloon
bonnet]! fye!
How daur ye do't?

O Jeany, dinna toss your head,
An set your beauties a' abread
[abroad]!
Ye little ken what cursed speed
The blastie's makin!

Thae winks an finger-ends, I dread,
Are notice takin!

O wad some Power the giftie gie us
To see oursels as ithers see us!
It wad frae [from] monie a blunder
free us
An foolish notion:

What airs in dress an gait wad lea'es
us,
An ev'n devotion!

Heads Up

There are three species of human lice: head, body, and crab (pubic) lice. Lice are ectoparasites, which means they infest the surface of the body but do not invade tissues. Body lice, infesting the body but not the head, are closely related to and similar in appearance to head lice. Body lice are currently uncommon in the United States. Crab lice infest the pubic areas of the body and differ greatly in appearance from head and body lice. Crab lice are more common than body lice but less common than head lice in the United States today. Control of body and crab lice differs from that of head lice.

Yup, lice have always been with us human types, and it looks like they always will be. The ubiquitous head louse (*Pediculus humanus capitis*), the subject of this book, seems to be spreading at epidemic proportions. While the U.S. Centers for Disease Control does not routinely track head lice infestations (pediculosis), many school nurses, various nonprofit groups, some health departments, and the pharmaceutical companies do. And according to these sources, in the United States, anywhere from 12 to 25 million Americans, mostly children, will be scratching their heads from a head-louse in-

There are approximately 12 million cases of head lice in the United States each year.

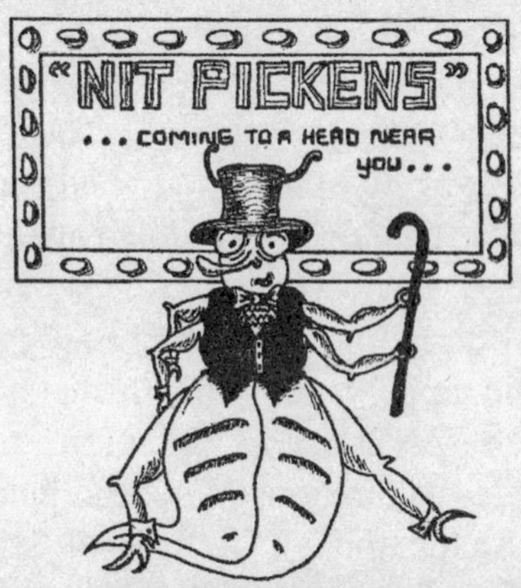

Heads Up

According to a 1997 article in the British *Sun News*, 65 percent of English schoolchildren have head lice.

festation this year alone. Worldwide, says C. V. Picollo and coauthors in a 1998 article in the *Entomological Society of America*, "the number of cases of head and body lice infestation has been estimated to be over 100 million."[1]

According to these statistics, head lice are more prevalent than chicken pox. In fact, head lice rival the common cold for the most common childhood ailment.

Heads Up

The *Los Angeles Times* of April 14, 1997, reports: "Ordinary lice may be turning into 'super lice,' developing immunity to over-the-counter treatments that are parents' chief weapons. A group of Israeli researchers said their tests have proved that head lice . . . are overpowering the over-the-counter treatments."

Who Gets Head Lice?

Rich, poor, royal or not, anyone can get head lice. The head louse is an equal opportunity parasite. Although school-age children get head lice more often than adults, girls slightly more than boys, the fact is that the pesky head louse can and does infest anyone. And now that head lice have become so difficult to get rid of, they are that much more likely to spread. Head lice don't like to be crowded. We like to think of them as pioneers, heading out to the wide, open spaces of the Old West to settle new territory. And they like clean, healthy heads the best! Wouldn't you?

Just think of the possibilities for migrating head lice! If a child gets head lice by playing on the floor and touching heads with other children, and has it long enough,

Head lice like clean, healthy heads the best.

that child is likely to infest his siblings. Once the siblings have it, the parents will likely get it. The siblings can pass it on to their classmates and their teachers. Camp counselors can get it, and then it's in the high schools and college campuses. Just like one great, big, out-of-control snowball, rolling rapidly downhill. Pretty soon everyone gets a turn.

So, if your precious darling is sent home with head lice, don't be embarrassed. You are in excellent and, most likely, very clean company. Check out the fanciest private school in your area—it probably has the worst head-louse problem because the people there are least likely to admit it!

Why Do People Get So Upset About a Few Insects on the Head?

Well, nobody likes the idea of "bugs" on their head, especially ones that itch as much as head lice do. Sometimes children itch so much that they have a hard time concentrating. Thus the expression "nitwit!"

Besides, head lice are hard to get rid of, and they can be seriously disruptive to family, school, and work life. A head-louse infestation can make children irritable and cause parents to become exhausted, hysterical, and ashamed. And if that is not enough, head lice can cause finger-pointing in a community and rifts among friends. Most of these problems are caused by a lack of information, a problem this book will help to eliminate.

Managing a head-louse infestation also takes considerable time and effort. It involves shampooing, nit-picking, and housecleaning. Working parents can have a difficult time managing a head-louse infestation, especially if their employer will not or cannot give them the necessary time off from work to get the problem under control.

Some of the shame and embarrassment associated with head lice comes from a mistaken confusion with body lice, a whole different animal. Body lice lay their eggs in the seams of clothing and bedding (as in bedbugs). They are spread by crowded conditions associated with poverty and the inability to wash and dry clothes and bed linen. In the United States today, body lice are usually found only on itinerant people or the homeless. However, we have encountered a few cases where callers have described finding them on their mattresses.

When you tell your kids "Good night, sleep tight, don't let the bedbugs bite!" you're telling them to pull the sheets tight over the mattress so the body lice won't bite!

So, if you buy a used mattress or have guests who don't have high standards of hygiene, you may, in fact, encounter body lice. But body lice do not infest the head and do not lay eggs on the hair shafts, so it is easy to tell the difference.

Body lice were responsible for spreading epidemic typhus, especially during World War I. In fact, more people died of typhus during World War I than from bullets. One major reason we won World War II was because the Swiss invented DDT, which killed the body lice and kept Allied soldiers from catching typhus. Axis troops had no access to DDT.

The reason we bring this up is not to freak you out but to explain the confusion between head lice and body lice. Probably this confusion causes uninformed people to associate head lice with a lack of hygiene.

Meanwhile, it is important for everyone to remember that: ***Head lice are not life threatening, just annoying!***

Heads Up

Head lice:

- Like clean, healthy heads the best.
- Don't transmit diseases.
- Are nearly as common as the common cold.
- Anyone can get them.

Body lice:

- Can carry diseases.
- Are associated with conditions where clothing cannot be regularly washed and dried or from infested mattresses.
- Are uncommon in the US at the present time.

Got it?

Heads Up

Pediculicides are the insecticidal shampoos and creme rinses used to treat head lice. These products contain pesticides and should be used with caution.

Please, don't blame the person who gave your child head lice. Next time it might be your child who passes them along. And we all need to work together if we want to defeat these annoying insects.

PESTICIDES—THE REAL PROBLEM

Today the big problem related to head lice may be the chemicals used to treat them. Because most people want head lice off their heads sooner rather than later, they spend millions of dollars on louse treatment products. The makers of pediculicides (the chemicals used to treat head lice) take in over $150 million a year from assorted insecticidal louse shampoos, creme rinses, and sprays.

Any chemical that kills pests is a pesticide, and all pesticides have the potential to cause serious side effects. The general consensus among public health professionals is that people need to worry more about the pesticides they are pouring on their children's heads than about the lice themselves. And if parents are going to use pesticides on their children's heads, they need to check with their physician or pharmacist, to make sure the brand they choose is effective and safe for their child.

Why are there more head lice these days than there were twenty and thirty years ago?

Head lice are most often spread through head-to-head contact. Children, who are less inhibited than older people, tend to play together, tumbling around like puppies. These days children also go to school younger and remain for a longer time each day. They have more frequent and closer contact with other children outside their own families. Our classrooms are more open and children move around the class more freely instead of sitting quietly at separate desks. While this is great for kids' social and intellectual development, it also means kids are exposed to head lice and other childhood illnesses at a younger age.

According to the *Common Sense Pest Quarterly*, a surprisingly large number of people are willing to tolerate the existence of head lice on their heads. This may be a result of the increased amount of work and the difficulty involved in eliminating the infestation.

Another major culprit in the head-lice wars appears to be the rise of *new strains of chemically tolerant, pesticide-resistant head lice.*

For several years the media, mothers, school nurses, and entomologists have been

Heads Up

"We've been getting reports from school nurses from all over the country," said Terri Meinking, a University of Miami researcher who cowrote a 1986 report on head-lice treatment. "When they say it doesn't work the way it used to, we have to take that seriously."

reporting that *many head-louse populations have become resistant to the chemicals used to treat them.* (See Chapter 3.)

While some scientists and public health professionals doubt the existence of resistant head lice, anecdotal and scientific evidence about the growth of such strains is now overwhelming. A group of Israeli researchers claim that their tests show that head lice are definitely overpowering the chemicals used to treat them. And in April of 1998, *The Wall Street Journal* reported that a study by the Harvard School of Public Health determined that head lice appear to have developed resistance to permethrin, the active ingredient in Nix. Because the molecule in permethrin is almost identical to the molecule in pyrethrin, the active ingredient in Rid, Pronto, A200, and most other pediculicides, there is almost certain to be crossover resistance.

Reports of treatment failure when using Nix, Rid, and Clear (the most commonly used over-the-counter pediculicides) have been widespread and persistent despite assurances from the companies that their products are 99 to 100 percent effective. Indications are that prescription medications such as Kwell, whose active ingredient is the neurotoxin lindane, are also ineffective in eliminating many louse populations. (Lindane is toxic to humans and has been known to cause seizures, temporary paralysis, and death.)

Where once a single treatment of a pediculicide was sufficient to get rid of head lice, parents across the country now report treatment failure after multiple doses.

The idea of resistant head lice is not surprising. Living creatures are resilient. Over time they can become resistant to any chemical. Check out the long shelf life of cockroaches, bacteria, fire ants, mosquitoes, and the like. It seems that no matter what we humans do to control them, they just keep coming back for more.

Unfortunately, conflicting information over the existence of strains of pesticide-resistant head lice has caused tremendous

Heads Up

"Products that have been working aren't working anymore."—John Erdmann, entomologist, University of Massachusetts

confusion and frustration for parents. Depending on whom a parent talks to, the recommended treatments for a head-louse infestation can range from the ineffective to the potentially dangerous. And some of that misinformation can come from the medical establishment, which receives much of its information about head lice from the manufacturers of pediculicides.

In order to protect children's health, parents and health professionals would be wise to adopt a conservative approach when dealing with head lice.

Why should you stay away from the chemical warfare approach?

There may be a few doubting Thomases or very frustrated parents who, when confronted with head lice on their children, say, "I don't care, just give me drugs, lots of them." It's the old chemical warfare, "a pill for every purpose" or "better living through chemistry" approach. The problem with the chemical warfare approach is that we are dealing with children. No long-term studies have proven that repeated doses of most insecticides on children's scalps are safe. In fact, the BBC recently reported that children's scalps are more absorbent than previously believed and that pesticides are eliminated from their bodies more slowly.

If you are tempted to ignore long-term health concerns and do decide to give the chemical warfare (applying multiple doses of pediculicides) approach a try, think about this as well: The chemical warfare approach doesn't seem to be very effective. The authors have personally talked to thousands of parents who have used pediculicides six or seven times and still find live lice on their children's heads.

We are not suggesting that a pediculicide, used as directed by the manufacturer, can't be part of an effective treatment program to rid your child of a head-louse infestation. But in the case of pediculicides, stronger or more often is not better. Exceeding the recommended dose or increasing the amount of time you leave a pediculicide on the head does not increase your chances of eliminating head lice, but it might compromise your child's health. So don't let this little creature freak you out so much that you lose your common sense when it comes to health matters.

Heads Up

According to the U.S. Environmental Protection Agency, "All pesticides are toxic to some degree, this means they can pose a risk to you, to your children and pets. . . ."

Use caution with pediculicides and be aware that there are safer and easier ways to get rid of head lice then turning your child's scalp—and your own—into a chemical dumping ground.

But if you feel you must try a pediculicide, be aware that head-louse infestations usually cause itching and scratching. Therefore, it is important to check each person's head carefully for open wounds before applying any chemical. Never use a pediculicide on anyone with cuts, abrasions, or inflammation. Follow the three steps listed below for specific guidelines on how to apply pediculicides safely.

Three Steps to Follow When You Feel You Must Use a Pediculicide

1) Make sure that your child actually has head lice before you treat with pediculicides. Misdiagnosis of head lice occurs more often than you think. Do not treat unless you

Heads Up
Never use pediculicides on infants under six months of age or if you are pregnant or nursing.

see nits (tiny oval eggs attached at an angle to one side of the hair shaft) or live lice. And never use a pediculicide as a preventive.

2) Check with your pharmacist and use only an over-the-counter pediculicide appropriate and safe for each member of your family. Follow the manufacturer's dose and application directions exactly. Never apply any products containing lindane (Kwell), a powerful neurotoxin with the potential for serious side effects.
3) Be prepared to take additional (nonchemical) steps to get rid of those head lice that have developed resistance to the pediculicide. There is an excellent chance that the pediculicide will not kill all the lice, and it takes only one pregnant louse or two amorous ones to create a whole new generation of head lice.

What exactly does a pesticide-resistant head louse mean to an itchy public?
If resistant head lice are on the rise, as many experts now believe, schools and par-

Heads Up

According to a 1998 article in *Consumer Reports*, "The Consumer's Union petitioned the FDA [Food and Drug Administration] to outlaw this [Lindane] neurotoxic, possibly carcinogenic pesticide as a lice treatment sixteen years ago."

ents may have to deal with widespread and difficult-to-contain infestations. Parents will need to take a deep breath and realize that there are no more overnight solutions to the problem of head lice. Schools will have to plan ahead in order to prevent schoolwide infestations. And everyone will have to avoid blaming others for not containing the problem.

However, encountering resistant head lice does not mean that families have to live with them. A case of resistant head lice simply means that people cannot rely on a quick chemical fix. Instead, families and schools will have to follow an integrated, multistep treatment protocol like the Five-Step Battle Plan outlined in this book to get rid of head lice.

Yikes, we can hear the groans all over America. "What do you mean I can't just shampoo my kid's head and wake up when it's all over?"

Sorry, folks, the days of wham, bang, shampoo your head, ma'am, the wicked lice are dead are past. New treatments are on the horizon, but they will take time to reach the drugstore. Even if these treatments do work, and they are proven to be safe enough to be approved by the Food and Drug Administration (FDA), it is almost inevitable that head lice eventually will become resistant to these new chemicals. And before we blithely pour these new pesticides on our children's heads, remember that it takes about twenty-five years to see the complete consequences of any new chemical. If a chemical kills lice on contact, what is it doing to our children? Is it worth the worry and guilt, when, with a little extra effort, we can eliminate head lice with a nontoxic treatment program that also happens to make your hair look fabulous? Call us crazy, but we believe this one is a no-brainer.

GOOD NEWS ABOUT HEAD LICE

Yes, Virginia, there is a Santa Claus. While head lice are adaptable and hard to get rid of, they are not invincible. You don't need a nuclear bomb to treat them. You just need to arm yourself with a few basic facts and outsmart these persistent critters. By learning what head lice and their eggs look like, understanding how they operate and proliferate, and following sensible treatment and prevention steps, you can make sure these annoying creatures go away and do not come back to play another day.

Wading through all this information may seem like a lot of work, but the alternative could be a battle with head lice that lasts for months or even years. Weigh the cost of becoming a louse expert with the cost of lost work days, missed school days, and thousands of dollars spent on chemicals and dry cleaning. We have had people tell us that they have spent over $2,000 on shampoos, louse sprays, combs, and cleaning services. Then they call us hysterical because they still have head lice.

So if head lice have invaded your nest, think war. Lock and load by arming yourself with the basic facts about head lice. Prepare for battle against "the creepin blastit wonner."

KNOW YOUR ENEMY!

What are head lice?

Very simply, the head louse is an ectoparasitic, blood-sucking parasite from the insect order *Anoplura*. It is adapted to live on the human scalp and neck. About the size of a sesame seed (or smaller), head lice can range in color from light brown to dark gray or black. They have six legs which all end in claws, are wingless, and burrow their mouthparts into the scalp to feed once or more each day.

Head lice have three growth stages—nit (egg), nymph (larva), and adult.

Where do head lice come from?

Head lice do not live in the air or the dirt; they live on human scalps. Dead lice have even been found on prehistoric mummies. Lice probably will be around as long as there are humans to act as hosts.

While some scientists speculate that lice may have come from monkeys, others say humans gave lice to monkeys!

However, household pets do not transmit their lice to us, and we cannot give our lice to our pets. So don't use treatments meant for human on your pets and vice versa.

What is a louse's life cycle?

A louse lives around thirty days. It takes eight to ten days for an egg to hatch and another eight to ten days for a louse to mature enough to lay eggs of its own. During the eight-to-ten-day maturation process, the young nymphs molt three times, growing larger with each molt. The nymphs are very hard to see because they are very nearly transparent and only about the size of a pe-

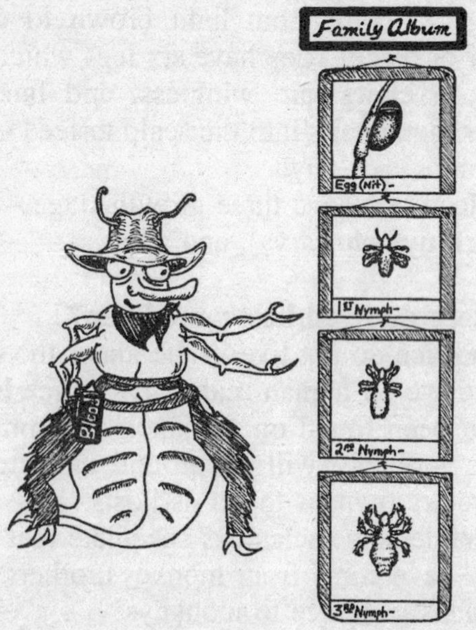

Heads Up

The louse is approximately 2.4 to 3.3 mm long.

riod. Adult lice move very quickly on a hair shaft and are hard to see because they hide from the light. When you part the hair to take a look, they've already moved on. That's why most people diagnose a head-louse infestation by finding nits.

A mature louse lays about six eggs a

Heads Up
People generally get head lice through direct contact with an infested person. Head-to-head contact is the most common way to spread head lice.

day. When dealing with a head-louse infestation, you want to make sure to check for nits and remove them. The only way to know if you still have head lice is to remove all the nits, then see if you find more nits over the next ten days. If you do find more nits, you still have live lice on your head, whether you have seen them in their travels or not.

How do you get head lice?

No matter what anyone tells you, *head lice cannot hop, jump, or fly.* While they can crawl fairly quickly on a hair shaft, once a louse is off the head, it is strictly slow motion. If you see a creature jumping or flying off a head, it is not a louse.

What is vector transmission?

There is some disagreement among entomologists and other experts about whether head lice are commonly spread through vectors—that is, through an infested persons' belongings, such as brushes, combs, hats, jackets, and to a lesser extent towels, pillows, and earphones.

In England, entomologists say vectors cannot spread head lice. Therefore, they do not feel that it is necessary to do any cleaning as part of a program to eliminate an infestation. English health officials felt our video *Head Lice to Dead Lice* emphasized cleaning the environment too much, and they chose not to endorse the video on that basis. Health officials there were concerned that if they told people to clean, they might focus on cleaning and using louse sprays instead of on their heads. However, according to an article in the British *Sun News*, 65 percent of English schoolchildren are infested with head lice. And England even has a National Bug Busting Day to encourage everyone to attack that country's burgeoning head-louse epidemic at the same time. Also, we have received letters from many parents and nurses in England desperate for advice on how to control their widespread problem. All this makes us believe there may be a problem with English entomologists' confidence that vector transmission is impossible. (See Chapter 7 for a differing opinion from Mary Ward, professional nit-picker, who has treated thousands of children for head lice.)

Because lice can live off a human head

Heads Up

Lice can live off a human head for twenty-four to thirty-six hours. They live longer in warm, humid climates. One nitpicker reported watching a large louse survive for 72 hours.

for up to thirty-six hours, most entomologists and health professionals in the United States recommend a moderate cleaning program (see Chapter 3) to remove lice from the environment.

We suggest that people take a middle-of-the-road position regarding the possibility of vector transmission. Lice prefer human heads and don't live very long when they are off heads. So concentrate most of your lice removal efforts on heads. But for those hardy lice or nits that manage to land on a comb and stay alive for a while, a sensible and moderate program like the P-V-P program outlined in Chapter 3 should take care of the problem.

What are the symptoms of a head-louse infestation?

The most common symptom of a head-louse infestation is itching, primarily at the base of the neck, behind the ears, and at the crown of the head. The itching is

Heads Up
It often takes about a week before symptoms of a head-louse infestation appear.

caused by an allergic reaction to the saliva that head lice inject into the scalp to keep the bite opening from closing. People who are not allergic to the saliva never itch at all. Other people continue to itch even after the lice have been eliminated. After all, a mosquito bite doesn't stop itching just because the mosquito has flown away.

Repeat infestations can cause some people to become supersensitive to the bites. Individuals experiencing persistent, intense itching and discomfort should visit a dermatologist.

More severe symptoms of head lice include swollen glands and a feeling of malaise, hence the term "nitwit." And people may easily get a secondary bacterial infection from the scratching. This should come as no surprise. We all know that children don't always wash their hands before they scratch an itch. Any infections that result should be treated under a physician's supervision.

Because symptoms of an infestationn may not show up right away, it's a good idea to check your child's head every day for a couple of weeks if your child has been exposed to head lice.

How do you check for head lice?

Diagnosis of head lice is usually made by finding lice eggs (nits). Nits are tiny, oval, yellow or gray translucent eggs firmly attached to one side of the hair shaft at an angle. If you can blow or flick it off, it is not a nit.

Viable nits are usually, but not always, found within a half inch of the scalp. The mother louse lays the eggs close to the scalp to provide warmth. In warmer climates or seasons, you are more likely to see viable eggs farther from the scalp.

To check for nits, use natural or other bright light. Look all through the head, particularly behind the ears, at the crown, and at the back of neck. Check the scalp for lice as well as nits. A magnifying glass can be helpful, particularly for those people with over-forty eyes. Make sure you do a thorough head check because lice and nits can be difficult to find.

You can also comb through the hair with a nit comb. If you are an adult and have no one to help you look, Lennie Copeland, author of *The Lice-Buster Book*, recommends that you comb over a white towel, making sure to catch everything that falls.

Heads Up

If you have to pull a suspected nit the whole length of the hair shaft to get it off, and it doesn't crumble in your fingers, it is probably a nit.

Use your magnifying glass to make a correct diagnosis of head lice. If you see something moving, and it's not flying or jumping, look closely to determine if it is a louse.

People who have been treated for lice over a long period of time can develop DEC (desquamated epithelial cell) plugs. These plugs consist of oil produced by the scalp to compensate for excessive dryness caused by the treatment. They are white, greasy clumps stuck to a hair shaft. You can tell them from nits because they usually stick all the way around the hair shaft instead of being attached at an angle to one side.

People also mistake hair casts (dandruff) and hair spray droplets for nits. But as we said, if it comes off easily or flakes off, it is not a nit.

How do you get rid of head lice?

Getting rid of head lice is a three-step process. *First, you must kill all the nymphal and adult lice.* This can be tricky business in the age of pesticide resistance. Pediculicides can no longer be relied on to do the complete job. But if you don't get rid of these adult lice, you could be nit-picking forever, a tiresome occupation. That's why using olive oil treatments to smother lice or slow them down enough to be caught in a nit comb is proving to be a safe and effective treatment option for many families. (For a complete list of louse-killing methods, read Chapter 2.)

Second, manually remove all nits and continue to check frequently and thoroughly for nits over a twenty-one-day period—the life cycle of the head louse. This is a critical step. Experts agree that if you skip this step, you could be battling your head-louse infestation for a very long time. (See Chapter 4 for a good description of this process.)

Third, you should do a reasonable, but not obsessive job, of cleaning the home environment. See Chapter 3 for the P-V-P method of housecleaning.

How do I know if I am louse free?

You have managed to get rid of a head-louse infestation if your child is nit free for ten to twelve days straight. That means you, as a parent, have to be responsible to check for and remove nits. You should not expect the school nurse or another child to do this job.

Remember that getting rid of head lice takes time and effort. The more you know, the faster you will get rid of them. And don't forget to smile!

2

The Thrill of the Kill

Getting Rid of Head Lice—Chemical Treatments, Smothering Techniques, Folk Remedies, and Manual Removal

First do no harm.

The treatments for head lice are probably as old as the creature itself, and they range from comic to dangerous (like the use of kerosene). An eleven-year-old girl in Boston was hospitalized with burns over 30 percent of her body when the gasoline her parents used to kill her head lice was ignited by a nearby stove. That being said, here is a treatment listed in Herb Walker's *Country Store*, which lists old remedies, recipes, and advertisements. **Do not try this**:

Heads Up

The definition of a pesticide, according to the Office of Prevention, Pesticides and Toxic Substances, is "Any substance or mixture of substances intended for preventing, destroying, repelling or mitigating any pest."

> Lice, to Get Rid of Them: First, put your clothes on an anthill. Then wash your head in kerosene. Sprinkle your head with ocean salt and then, parting the hair, pour raw whisky on your scalp. Let it stay for 48 hours. Do not smoke or go near the fire.

The booklet also lists the following as the cure for baldness:

> Smear your head with fresh cow manure.

Please don't go spreading that suggestion around either. There are probably a lot of guys out there vain and desperate enough to try it.

Throughout recent history, people have used a wide range of products to cure head lice, including malathion, DDT, coal oil, kerosene, and pet sprays. You name it, people seem to have tried it, and that's the problem—sometimes the cure is worse than the lice.

Today many people in North America use

over-the-counter creme rinses and shampoos called pediculicides to kill head lice. Calling these products creme rinses and shampoos is somewhat misleading because they are really pesticides, and all pesticides can have side effects. Many pesticides have been associated with an increased risk of cancer, birth defects and reproductive disorders. The terms "creme rinse" or "shampoo" sound more benign and improve sales, but it doesn't change the fact that the product is a pesticide.

We are surrounded by pesticides. They are in our food supply, homes, yards, water, and air. According to the Environmental Protection Agency's Office of Prevention, Pesticides and Toxic Substances, "About 2.2 billion pounds of pesticides are used annually in the U.S." Even though any pesticide designed for use on humans must undergo rigorous testing by the Food and Drug Administration before it is approved, it is prudent to limit exposure to pesticides as much as possible. Use your common sense and act cautiously when you decide to apply products that contain pesticides to yourself or your children.

Pediculicidal products are considered pesticides, and they are generally the first line of defense in the war against head lice. The authors would like to say that we do not think these products are absolutely necessary to get rid of a head-lice infestation, and, in general, we

Heads Up

According to Attorney General Vasco of New York State, Children are more sensitive than adults to many toxic chemicals, including pesticides. Some toxins will damage children's growing and developing tissues more readily than fully established adult tissues . . . Further, children taking medication may be at increased risk from pesticide exposure."

In 1998 Americans spent $159.5 million on head lice treatments

strongly recommend against using currently available prescription medications for head lice. We do not have a problem with people using over-the-counter pediculicides as long as they follow safe and proper guidelines:

- Never use pediculicides on pregnant or nursing mothers, or on infants under the age of six months.
- Check with your pharmacist or physician and choose the product that is appropriate and safe for each member of your family.
- Follow the directions on the package ex-

"The Dose Is the Poison"
Paracelcius

actly—never use more than what is recommended.

- Never use these products on eyebrows or eyelashes.
- Do not use a pediculicide if you have cuts or abrasions on the skin or scalp.
- Use recommended precautions when applying the pediculicide.
- Discontinue use of a pediculicide if it is not working.
- Recognize that none of these products is 100 percent effective, and additional steps, such as manual nit-picking, will be necessary to end a head-louse infestation.
- Avoid any products containing lindane or malathion. Malathion is currently banned for use on humans in the United States but available in Europe.
- See a physician if you have an allergic reaction.

When you apply any of these products, remember that they are for external use only. You do not want these products to get into your eyes or into your mucous membranes (nose, mouth, or vagina). Avoid inhaling them. Apply the products over the sink, not in the tub or shower. And be aware that children's scalps and lungs can be highly sensitive. Rinse the product off immediately if your child complains of a burning scalp or has trouble breathing. Call your physician immediately if you are concerned about a reaction to a pediculicide.

CHEMICAL TREATMENTS

OVER-THE-COUNTER PEDICULICIDES: USE CAUTION!

Here's what you have to evaluate when you are considering using a chemical treatment: The lice on your child's head may or may not be of a resistant strain. If your child has contracted a nonresistant domestic strain or has contracted head lice from someone who came from a country that has not overused a particular pediculicide, the lice may, in fact, succumb or at least partially succumb to that pediculicide. However, if you use a specific pediculicide once and it doesn't work, using it again won't help.

Although many populations of head lice have developed resistance to these products, pediculicides still can be helpful as one step in a multifaceted head louse treatment program like the Five-Step Battle Plan.

> Louse product earnings increased 8.1 percent in 1998 alone.

PYRETHRINS (RID, PRONTO, A-200, BARC, R&C)

Pyrethrins are insecticides derived from the chrysanthemum flower. They are combined with piperonyl butoxide, a synergist agent that boosts the power of pyrethrins. Piperonyl butoxide has been banned in the United Kingdom because of its chemical instability. Pyrethrins have limited residual activity; they require a second treatment (seven to ten days later). They are meant to kill crawling lice and have no effect on nits (louse eggs), so they have to be reapplied in case some nits are not removed and hatch on the head.

Pyrethrins may cause reactions in individuals allergic to ragweed pollen or chrysanthemums. Although these reactions are not common, such individuals should not use any product containing pyrethrin. Anyone who decides to use a pyrethrin should read the label and FDA warnings carefully before applying this product.

Treatment failure with pyrethrins is common today.

PERMETHRIN (NIX)

Permethrin is synthetic pyrethrin; its molecules are very similar to those of pyrethrin. People who have allergic reactions to pyrethrins may also be allergic to permethrin. Warner Lambert developed permethrin and markets it under the name Nix.

According to the directions on the box, permethrin products require only a single dose, although the manufacturers of Nix say that you can apply another dose if you see live lice a week or more after first applying the product. Permethrin leaves a residue on the hair and supposedly has residual lice-killing activity for another week or so. When first marketed, this residue killed the newly hatched nymphs, thus making a second application unnecessary. Permethrins are considered to be more effective than pyrethrins and less toxic because they are not readily absorbed by the skin. Permethrin and pyrethrin molecules are so similar that some entomologists say if lice are resistant to one, they probably will also be resistant to the other.

The Harvard School of Public Health performed a study to demonstrate whether some head-louse populations had developed resistance to permethrin and, by association, pyrethrin.

On April 1, 1998, *The Wall Street Journal* reported that "A Harvard University Research team has confirmed a widely held suspicion that some head lice in the U.S. are now resistant to permethrin, the leading treatment for louse infestation . . ."

Individuals using Nix should read the label

before applying the product. According to the manufacturer, permethrin-based products can cause breathing difficulties in susceptible persons.

Some physicians, pharmacists, or written information on head lice recommend leaving permethrin products on longer than the directions indicate. We believe this is unwarranted, possibly unsafe, and may be a factor contributing to the growth of resistant head lice.

Treatment failure with permethrin products is now widespread.

PRESCRIPTION MEDICATIONS: RARELY NECESSARY

LINDANE

Consumer Reports and the Environmental Protection Agency believe that lindane (Kwell) should be taken off the market for use on humans. In fact, lindane has already been banned in eighteen countries. The 1997 *Physician's Red Book* states that according to a Report of the Committee on Infectious Disease of the American Academy of Pediatrics, lindane is "contraindicated for premature infants, persons with known seizure disorders, and those with hypersensitivity to the product, and should be used with caution in patients with inflamed or traumatized skin and in pregnant or nursing women."

We do not believe that this is a strong enough warning. Lindane is a powerful neurotoxin that can have serious side effects, such as seizures, rashes, leukemia, temporary paralysis, and possibly death, if it is accidentally ingested or misused. At the American Head Lice Information Center (a public service provided by Sawyer Mac Productions), we have received several phone calls from elderly grandparents who used lindane on their grandchildren. Several reported vomiting blood after applying the product. According to a 1995 publication on pest mangagement by the attorney general's office in New York, "The elderly may have heightened sensitivity to pesticides as a result of the natural decline of various body systems which occurs with age."

Besides being expensive, more toxic, and a higher risk, lindane does not appear to be any more effective (because of resistance) than other less-toxic medications, and it must be left on for a longer period of time. Therefore, there is no reason to consider using lindane. Unfortunately, many physicians who are not acquainted with its hazards or nontoxic alternatives still prescribe lindane when parents complain that over-the-counter lice-killing medications aren't working. We believe the American Medical Association and the American Pediatric Association should counsel physicians against prescribing lindane for the treatment of head lice.

For your family's safety, make sure you do not use any product containing lindane.

MALATHION

Malathion, an organophosphate, is a cousin to nerve gas. It is used in the United States for agricultural purposes but has been banned for use on humans. Malathion can burn the eyes and has a strong odor. It is a popular medication in other countries because it is considered to have strong louse-killing properties, and it is less toxic than lindane.

According to Extoxnet, the Extension Toxicology Network:

> It has been reported that single doses of malathion may affect immune system response. Symptoms of acute exposure to organophosphate or cholinesterase-inhibiting compounds may include the following: numbness, tingling sensations, incoordination, headache, dizziness, tremor, nausea, abdominal cramps, sweating, blurred vision, difficulty breathing or respiratory depression and slow heartbeat. Very high doses may result in unconsciousness, incontinence and convulsions or fatality.

You have to leave malathion on for eight to twelve hours and repeat the dose nine days later if you see signs of live lice.

Resistance to malathion also appears to be growing, particularly in England, where the drug has been in use for twenty-five years.

We certainly do not recommend using a drug that the U.S. Food and Drug Administration has banned for use on humans.

IVERMECTIN

Stromectol (ivermectin) is a semisynthetic derivative of the avemectin class of highly active broad-spectrum antiparasitic agents. The oral version, which is primarily donated by Merck Pharmaceuticals for use in Africa, is highly effective for the treatment of river blindness and an intestinal parasite. The topical version is not approved for use on humans.

Researchers have begun to test ivermectin's potential as a treatment for head lice and scabies, but at this time it is not approved as a treatment for either problem on humans.

Some physicians have begun to prescribe ivermectin as a head-louse treatment. However, studies have not yet been released to the public as to its effectiveness. Even if ivermectin proves to be effective, it is unlikely that it will be 100 percent effective, which means that anyone who uses it will still have to manually pick nits and use a smothering agent like olive oil.

The decision to use ivermectin or any chemical for an off-label use should be made only as a last resort and after careful research and consultation with a physician.

What does the future hold?

In all likelihood, the future holds many new products for head lice. There will always be some risk in using any pesticide. The FDA approves such products on a risk/benefit ratio. Unfortunately, it takes twenty-five years to get total information on risk. The FDA approval process takes only two years. But when you're dealing with children, twenty-five years brings them into the years of young adulthood and parenthood. It's in all of our best interests to keep the risks to our children as low as possible.

Use your common sense when it comes to making decisions about these products. So far we are not overly impressed with the track records of many large corporations when it comes to revealing product information that might result in reduced sales. You're the parent. You and your family must bear the ultimate risk. Do your own risk/benefit analysis.

SMOTHERING AGENTS

SAFE AND EFFECTIVE WHEN USED PROPERLY

Head lice breathe through holes in their sides called spiracles. When those holes are covered for long enough, lice will suffocate and die. However, head lice can hold their breath for hours, so using a smothering agent to get rid of head lice requires that the agent be left on for a significant amount of time, and coverage needs to be fairly complete to be successful. Using a smothering agent can be a good option for individuals who cannot or do not wish to use chemical treatments or who wish to supplement their chemical program as insurance against resistance and reinfestation.

OLIVE OIL

The authors believe that olive oil is the safest and most effective smothering agent available for head lice. Olive oil is nontoxic (except to a relatively few individuals who are allergic to olives), easy to apply, and washes out of the hair quickly.

According to the Common Sense Pest Control Quarterly, published by the Bio-Integral Resource Center, a nonprofit corporation formed in 1979 to provide practical information on the least-toxic methods for managing pests,

"Straight chain fatty acids with carbon chains of 10 and 18 atoms have been shown to be particularly useful as insecticides. Such fatty acids are found in coconut and olive oils."

Dr. Richard Pollack, an entomologist at the Harvard School of Public Health, has told the authors that "Any insect will succumb to anoxia (lack of oxygen) after being submerged in oil for a prolonged period." We asked Dr. Pollack to perform some informal laboratory tests on olive oil. (See Harvard Letter in appendix.) The tests confirmed that after being submerged in olive oil for several hours, head lice succumbed to anoxia.

However, the human scalp is not a petri dish. So the authors, with the assistance of professional nit-picker Mary Ward, tried several protocols on families with head lice before settling on the treatment method outlined in Chapter 4.

To be effective, smothering must be done correctly. The oil must be left on the hair for at least eight hours. The hair must be combed with a good metal nit comb with the smothering agent still on the hair. And the olive oil protocol must be repeated on specific days in the life cycle of the louse in order to remove lice that have hatched from any nits that were missed. Infested scalps must be carefully monitored for a full three weeks.

Many uninformed sources or those selling their own lice products claim that the use of olive oil to suffocate head lice is an old wives' tale. But the use of oil to smother lice is based on well-known and widely accepted scientific principles. The authors have received thousands of phone calls from grateful mothers, school nurses, pediatricians, and public health officials attesting to the success of this nontoxic treatment program.

It only takes a little common sense to realize how and why oil works. Any animal that requires oxygen to survive will die if denied oxygen for a sufficient period of time. The fact is, we have yet to hear of a case where people used olive oil correctly and failed to eliminate the infestation.

Olive oil should be considered as the first treatment of choice for head lice and as a backup to chemical treatments. It's cheap, effective, and nontoxic. In our experience, the final results are the same between people who choose to use the olive oil in conjunction with a pediculicide and those who choose to use only the olive oil.

The olive oil protocol does require time and persistence, so it may not be for everyone. And, as with all treatments for head lice, the olive oil protocol requires manual nit-picking to remove the eggs. The authors' 15-minute video, *Head Lice to Dead Lice: Safe Solutions for Frantic Families*, visually demonstrates how to use olive oil as part of a Five-Step Battle Plan to get rid of head lice.

What about other oils?
Other oils, such as baby, safflower, corn, peanut, and coconut oil, probably can also be used. But we know of no tests performed with these oils. People who are allergic to peanuts (or any of the other products) obviously should not use that product to smother lice. And mineral oil can cause muscle cramps and damage mucous membranes.

What about butter and mayonnaise?
Some people use butter or mayonnaise as smothering agents. However, they are much more likely to grow bacteria than oil products and are difficult to wash out of the hair. No protocol has been developed for determining the length, timing, and number of treatments. We do not recommend their use.

What about Vaseline?
Vaseline has been used to smother head lice, but it is extremely difficult to get out of the hair. Because nit-checking and removal should be done on clean, dry hair, Vaseline makes these actions tedious and often ineffective. Therefore, while it may smother adult lice, Vaseline actually does

Heads Up

People have used olive oil to prevent dandruff and wrinkles, soften the skin, reduce the effects of alcohol, control high blood pressure, condition hair and nails, and clear acne.

Heads Up

Just because something is natural doesn't mean it's safe.

not work well to eliminate the infestation in the long run. Dr. Terry Meinking, who originally supported the use of Vaseline, said in a phone conversation with the authors that she has come to regret her recommendation because Vaseline is so difficult to remove.

FOLK REMEDIES

EFFECTIVE, INEFFECTIVE, DANGEROUS

Throughout history people have used folk remedies to cure a variety of ailments.

Many of our most toxic poisons are completely "natural." If you want to have serious nightmares, read about these "natural poisons" in *Deadly Doses, a Writer's Guide to Poisons* by Serita Deborah Stevens with Anne Klarner. Check out what it says about the azalea, the delicious Barbados nut, belladonna, curare, hemlock, Jimsonweed, Lilies of the valley, oleander, rhododendron, summer snowflake, and English yew, all listed as "quickly fatal." In fact, you only have to drink the water that Lilies of the valley have been kept in and you will die.

Even some herbs, like nutmeg (a hallucinogen), which can be safely ingested in small quantities, can be dangerous in larger amounts. And don't forget, children's scalps are especially absorbent.

Be advised that most folk remedies have never been tested by scientists for safety or effectiveness against head lice. Caution should be the byword when dealing with any of these methods.

VINEGAR

While there is little evidence that vinegar is an effective remedy for killing head lice, a great deal of anecdotal evidence suggests that vinegar may be useful in nit removal. Because vinegar (apple cider and white), is comparatively harmless, we see no harm in using it to help loosen nits. Personally we have not seen it work, and consulting entomologists say that it is generally ineffective, but many people swear by it. Vinegar may be irritating to the eyes, so make sure to cover the eyes when applying it.

ESSENTIAL OILS (TEA TREE, PENNYROYAL, EUCALYPTUS, ROSEMARY)

The difference between these oils and olive oil is their potential for allergic reactions. Joan Sawyer used a tea tree oil shampoo during her louse infestation, and it burned her eyes and scalp so badly she was afraid she had done permanent damage. Some people have claimed success with tea tree oil, but we think it is too risky and irritating to try on children. Lennie Copeland, in her informative *The Lice-Buster Book*, does list a couple of recipes using essential oils to treat head lice. We suggest you use caution here! Pennyroyal has been known to cause miscarriage, and ylang ylang oil is not recommended for use in pregnant or nursing mothers. Why pay for these expensive oils or risk dangerous reactions? The FDA probably should regulate some of these oils.

GASOLINE OR KEROSENE

Both gasoline and kerosene were common treatments for head lice during World Wars I and II among soldiers and people on the home front. That's probably why both keep surfacing as a treatment for head lice. One problem is that gasoline and kerosene are incredibly flammable,

Heads Up
No comb alone will get rid of your head-lice infestation.

and many people have been horribly burned as a result of their use. Also, both are toxic and can be absorbed through the skin. In this day and age, there is no reason to consider trying something as dangerous as gasoline or kerosene. They should be avoided under any circumstance.

MANUAL REMOVAL

Picking out nits by hand is an essential part of any head lice treatment plan. However, relying solely on manual removal to get rid of adult head lice without the use of olive oil to slow them down probably will lead to frustration.

In addition to manual nit-picking, you also will need to use a nit comb (for a review of nit combs, see Chapter 4) to help with nit and lice removal.

LOUSE REMOVAL TOOLS

If you want to invest in only one lice removal tool, a good metal nit comb is best for removing both lice and nits. We recommend the metal ones because they are stronger, last longer, and some of them can be boiled. The all-plastic ones commonly end up with teeth missing, and that doesn't help you in your eradication efforts.

Lice are capable of getting away from any lice comb, unless they are covered with oil and their systems are slowed down. One organization that disparages the use of olive oil suggests instead that more than one person comb a child's hair at the same time in order to chase the lice. This seems to us inefficient, overly intimidating to the child, and a waste of valuable man- or womanpower. It's hard enough to find one person with the time and patience to pick nits. An army seems excessive. And frankly, we have a difficult time visualizing this procedure. But feel free to try it.

There are some other interesting items on the market to help get rid of head lice. Their effectiveness has yet to be established.

- *The Robi Comb*: This is a battery-powered comb that electrocutes the lice. It works sort of like a bug zapper. The problem is that there is a certain amount of risk to applying electricity to your child's scalp, and the Robi Comb can't be used with wet or oily hair. Entomologists have informed us that it reacts to debris in the hair as well as lice. We feel it is not the best choice.
- *The Nit Stripper*: This is a newly patented item that is designed like a surgical instru-

ment. It resembles a scissors with flat surfaces instead of blades. You slide a section of hair through it and it's supposed to strip off the nits. Unfortunately, we've only seen an early prototype, and parents complained that it pulled the hair and was awkward to use. The inventor has assured us that his product has been improved. It you have an enormous number of nits, the final incarnation of this may be an effective tool. But again, it will not take the place of a comb because it will not remove adult lice or nymphs from the scalp. So, if you are planning to buy only one tool, you're best off with a good metal nit comb. If you are into gadgets, you can check this out and let us know what you think.

The National Pediculosis Association (NPA) suggests using Scotch tape to catch lice on the scalp. This seems much more difficult, time consuming, and ineffective than using the olive oil to paralyze them and then combing them out. Children may object to the tape sticking to their hair and pulling. And with this method, there's no way to assure that you have found and eliminated all the lice.

3

The P-V-P Housecleaning Method—You Don't Have to Go Postal!

Your child has just been sent home with head lice. Or worse, it's bedtime and your child says his head is itchy. Your heart starts to pound, but you are, after a all, a responsible mother. So you look, and there they are—the dreaded nits. After you have quelled the hysteria by reminding yourself that head lice do not make people seriously sick, your first urge is to start frantically cleaning the house. Don't do it! Turning into an obsessive-compulsive cleaner will only exhaust you and freak your children out. Your house may get clean, but you will not get rid of head lice.

Before you take another step, make sure that you are seeing lice. Check by blowing or flicking at the suspected nit. If it comes off easily, it is not a nit. Nits are attached at an angle to one side of a hair shaft. If you pull a suspected nit along the hair shaft and it doesn't crumble,

What Leonardo DiCaprio said about head lice before he boarded the *Titanic*: "We're Americans. We don't get head lice."

it probably is a nit. If you are fairly convinced that you are dealing with a head-louse infestation, get that olive oil on everyone's head—*before* you use up all your energy cleaning your house.

As we stated in Chapter 1, some entomologists think that cleaning the house may even be a waste of time. For example, Dr. Richard Pollack, of the Department of Immunology and Infectious Diseases at the Harvard School of Public Health, states on his Head Lice Information web page, "Steps to clean lice from the house or washing or vacuuming will result in a cleaner house, but are unlikely to significantly reduce the infestation." This is most likely true, given that lice can't live very long off a human head (about thirty-six hours). And nits, once hatched, need a human blood meal within forty-five minutes to survive at all. The chances are remote that either an adult louse or a newly hatched nit will find its way to someone's head.

But here's the rub: It could happen. Especially if that louse or nit is laying in wait in a place where people frequently put their heads. So what's a conscientious mom, dad, and/or sig-

Heads Up
If you decide to boil your all-metal combs, make sure you keep your eye on the stove!

nificant other to do? Simple—clean the high-risk areas but don't make yourself crazy.

Follow our P-V-P cleaning plan, and you will have eliminated any stray lice or nits. And you won't have driven yourself or your family crazy in the process.

- P: Personal items first
- V: Vacuum the right stuff
- P: Planes, trains, and autos, etc.

STEP 1. P FOR PERSONAL ITEMS

If there are any stray lice or nits about, they are most likely attached to a hair shaft that has fallen on the infested person's personal items. So let's start with these.

COMBS AND BRUSHES

We recommend putting away all brushes, which are difficult to clean, and using combs for the next few weeks. You can buy new combs, or you can soak the old ones in hot water (150°F degrees centigrade) for twenty minutes. It is easy to see and remove stray hair on combs.

Check with the manufacturer about whether you can boil your plastic combs. You should make sure to clean all combs after each use during an infestation. And remember, *never share your combs, brushes, or hair ornaments with anyone, even members of your family.*

TOWELS

Run all towels through the dryer between uses. Towels used after showers or washing the hair are one of the most likely places to find lice.

CLOTHING

Take all the sweaters, hats, jackets, and coats used by the infested person within the last forty-eight hours and put them in a hot dryer for twenty to thirty minutes. Some people may feel compelled to wash these items, but according to most entomologists, washing clothes will only give you clean lice. The dryer is your best friend, because dry heat kills lice.

When your child comes home with head lice from camp, make sure that everything possible goes through the dryer. Sleeping bags and pillows can be dry-cleaned if they can't fit in the dryer. We do this when our kids come home from camp whether we see signs of head lice right away or not. (See Chapter 7.)

Drawstring laundry bags are handy items to keep around the house. Kids can take them to school and keep their extra clothes in them. They can also stuff their jackets and hats in them during a louse outbreak at school, and Mom can put the laundry bag and the clothes in the dryer at night.

Remember to hang family coats and jackets separately during an infestation. You don't want them to touch each other.

BEDDING

Again, use your common sense here. If you contracted head lice on vacation and have been away from the house for more than forty-eight hours, then you don't need to do anything about the bedding or anything else in the house.

If you have not been away, put the infested person's bedding in the dryer. Head lice are not likely to crawl all the way down the hall into another person's room.

Visually inspect pillowcases and pillows daily. If there is a louse or a hair, you will see it and can remove it. All you have to do with a louse is pick it up with a piece of Scotch tape, fold the tape over it, and put it in the wastebasket.

Summary: Whenever possible, dry clothes, bedding, and towels used in the past forty-eight hours by an infested person in the dryer for twenty minutes on a high setting.

STEP 2: V FOR VACUUMING THE HOUSE

Anything that can't be put in the dryer can be vacuumed, including stuffed animals. Some people like to pack up toys, stuffed animals, and Barbie dolls and put them away for two weeks. But vacuuming is much less disruptive to the child and equally as effective.

Vacuuming the house is probably a good idea. But don't feel like you have to get on all fours and vacuum every nook and cranny. After all, most children, unless they are direct descendants of Tom Thumb, are too big to hide under the sofa. If a hair shaft with a louse actually managed to find its way to the floor, the louse would then have to crawl across the floor, up the sofa, onto someone's clothes, and find its way to the scalp. Get the picture? A head louse with that level of mobility would qualify for an Olympic triathlon.

So, concentrate your vacuuming efforts on those rugs, sofas, and chairs where people rest their heads frequently and on any throw pillows that get a lot of use. Use a lint remover (the roller kind with the sticky tape) on hard-to-reach areas.

Do this step once and then stop. Concentrate on heads. As long as you continue with the olive oil and comb-outs on the required days, you should not have to clean your house again.

Summary: Vacuum rugs, sofa, and chairs where people rest their heads. It is only necessary to do this once.

STEP 3: PLANES, TRAINS, AND AUTOMOBILES

Think about all those heads pressed up against the upholstery of your family car. You can vacuum your car seats or you can run a lint remover over the seats. During the school year, when you are transporting kids back and forth, you might consider keeping a lint remover in your car. That way you can run it over the seats as a precaution. Again, use your common sense here, but remember that with head lice, an ounce of prevention goes a long way.

We take a lint remover along on plane and train trips now. Okay, we may look a little kooky, but since we started, our kids haven't gotten head lice. Uh-oh, now that we've said that, we'd better turn around three times and spit over our left shoulders to avoid the evil eye. Of course we're not superstitious, but why take chances?

Summary: Vacuum or use a lint remover on car seats. Use caution in movie theaters, trains, and planes.

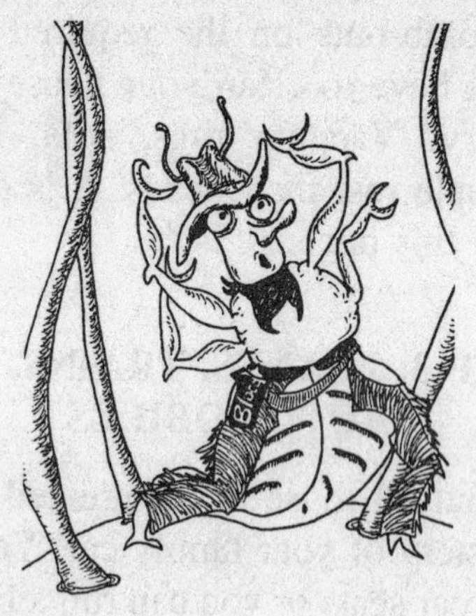

FEEL BETTER NOW?

If after reading this chapter, you still find yourself obsessed with cleaning, your fear of head lice and your feelings of being out of control have gotten the better of you. Take a deep breath and try to relax. The head lice will soon be gone and your life will return to normal.

4

Head Lice to Dead Lice: The Five-Step Battle Plan

The Five-Step Battle Plan, an integrated, safe approach to getting rid of head lice, is based on a treatment program first developed by a group of entomologists in Israel to eliminate head lice on their own children. These entomologists, who spent a lot of time dealing with pesticides, were very concerned about the dangers of using pesticides on young children. And in Israel, permethrin was made available ten years before it was available in the United States. Therefore, resistance began to develop there before it was recognized in the United States.

The Five-Step Battle Plan incorporates an integrated approach for the treatment of head lice. Dr. Richard Pollack, of the Harvard School of Public Health, states on his web page, "Success will likely depend on an integrated approach . . . combined with perseverance and a bit of levity."

Briefly, the five steps are:

1) Use a pediculicide (optional).
2) Apply olive oil treatment on *days 1, 5, 9, 13, 17, 21*. If you choose not to use a pediculicide, add *day 2* to the above list.
3) Clean the environment, following the P-V-P plan. (See Chapter 3.)
4) Comb out the lice and nits with the oil in the hair.
5) Check for nits regularly in clean, dry hair.

What you will need going into battle or what really smart parents have on hand *before* they get head lice:

- A great big bottle of the least expensive *olive oil* you can find. It doesn't have to be virgin; it doesn't have to be cold pressed. Pumace grade (olive oil in its crudest form) is actually best, if you can find it. This form is the least refined and contains more of the actual plant, which has many beneficial properties. Your local restaurant might sell you or your school a large can.
- A small plastic *applicator bottle* similar to the one used for applying color to hair.
- An over-the-counter pediculicide (if you choose to use one). Check with your physician or pharmacist for the one best suited for each member of your family. Remember, do not use anything containing Lindane (Kwell).
- Plastic shower caps.

- Bandannas.
- A good *metal nit comb* (see discussion of various nit combs on page 99).
- *Vision visor:* if you are visually challenged, you may want to consider getting one of these binocular magnifiers. They magnify two and a half times at 8" and help you see the nits while leaving your hands free to pick nits. They look like goggles and you can wear them with or without glasses. We find that wearing this gives us confidence in determining what we're seeing, especially since we are over forty. To order call 1-888-DIE LICE.
- A good clarifying shampoo like Clairol Herbal Essence Shampoo for Oily Hair or Prell.
- Covered elastic hair bands or hair clips to separate the hair.
- Clean white towels.
- Covered elastic bands or hair clips.
- Regular clean combs.

What you don't need are louse sprays—they're more harmful to your kids than the lice. The vacuum or lint remover work better.

THE FIVE-STEP BATTLE PLAN

STEP 1. USE AN OVER-THE-COUNTER PEDICULICIDE

This step is optional.

Remember, over the last several years, more

and more evidence has come to light that head lice are developing resistance to pediculicidal products. This is not surprising since insects usually develop resistance to pesticides. It's just a matter of time. There's a reason why cockroaches have been around longer than humans and probably will be around long after we're gone.

Whether you choose to use a pediculicide is a personal decision that should be made after consultation with your family physician. If you are uncomfortable using a pesticide, don't do it. You can still get rid of the lice. If, however, you feel compelled to do everything possible as quickly as possible to get them off your kids and out of your house, we feel it is acceptable to use an over-the-counter pediculicide. So, do what you have to do, as long as it's not dangerous to you or your child. If you use olive oil, you should be free of lice at the three-week mark, whether you chose to use a pediculicide or not.

Check with your physician to make sure that you or your child do not have allergies that will react to the pyrethrins, derivatives of the chrysanthemum (or to whatever other pediculicide has been selected).

STEP 2. THE OLIVE OIL TREATMENT

The olive oil treatment must be done on days 1, 5, 9, 13, 17, and 21. If you choose not to use a pediculicide, add day 2 to this list. These treat-

How to Use a Pediculicide

1. If you choose to use a permethrin or pyrethrin product, first wash the hair with a good clarifying shampoo like Prell to strip the hair of any other substances. Then dry the hair thoroughly. Using a pediculicide on wet hair will dilute the product.
2. Work at a sink, not in a tub or shower, so the pesticide goes only on the child's head. Cover the child's eyes with a wash cloth and use a full application. Apply the shampoo or creme rinse to dry hair, directly onto the scalp, and massage it through the hair and scalp thoroughly.
3. Using a timer, leave the pesticide on the head for the amount of time directed on the package and no longer. Wash it out, then go ahead and use a regular creme rinse or detangler. The package of Nix says other products interfere with the "residual effect" of permethrin, but since the residual effect may not work, make life easier for you and your child by making the hair easier to comb through.

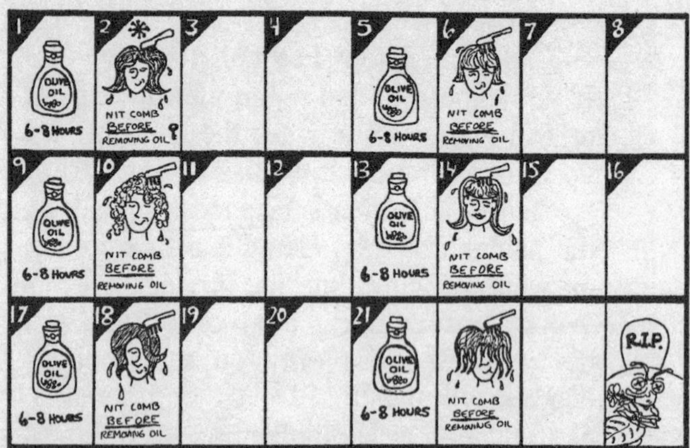

* IF YOU CHOOSE NOT TO USE A PEDICULICIDE, USE THE OLIVE OIL TREATMENT ON DAY 1 and DAY 2.

LEAVE THE OIL IN THE HAIR FOR THE COMB OUT. USING A GOOD METAL NIT COMB, COMB THE HAIR SECTION BY SECTION.

> Each female louse can lay up to 250 eggs during her 30-day life cycle.

ment days have been carefully chosen to disrupt the life cycle of the louse and maximize your chances of eliminating head lice. You must adhere to the exact treatment days to ensure successful completion of the program.

Using an applicator bottle, part the hair and apply the olive oil directly onto the scalp. Massage it in thoroughly, making sure to saturate the hair and scalp. Cover the head with a plastic shower cap, and keep it in place with a bandanna or bathing cap. If you use a bandanna, knot it at the top of the head where it won't

Heads Up
Rule of Thumb: Clean only slightly more than most people clean on a weekly basis.

interfere with sleeping. Leave the oil on for six to eight hours.

You may want to use a terry-cloth headband to absorb leakage.

Cover the pillow with a towel.

And while your kids are asleep with the olive oil quietly working its magic, it's time to move on to Step 3.

TIMING OF OLIVE OIL TREATMENTS

We spent a lot of time and effort determining the exact days on which to repeat the olive oil treatment. In order to make sure we found the best possible combination of treatment days, without exhausting families by requiring that they do more than necessary, our professional nit-picker, Mary Ward, worked with hundreds of families, trying different combinations of days. The goal, of course, was to ensure that every louse and nit was consistently eliminated by the three-week mark.

STEP 3. CLEAN THE ENVIRONMENT

This is one of the more controversial issues involving head lice. How much cleaning is necessary? See Chapter 3 for a full discussion.

Follow the P-V-P method outlined in Chapter 3: personal items first, then vacuum, then check your car and be careful in public places where your head rests against cloth seats (planes, trains, and movie theaters.)

STEP 4. THE COMB-OUT—COMB THOSE LICE RIGHT OUTTA YOUR HAIR

Please note that combing out lice and nits is an extremely important step in eliminating an infestation—perhaps the most important step of all. The few times people have had trouble eliminating the infestation using the Five-Step Battle Plan can almost always be traced to a failure to do this step correctly. Bear in mind that the olive oil does not kill head lice the way a pesticide does, on contact. Olive oil smothers the lice by covering holes in their sides called spiracles, through which the lice breathe oxygen.

However, head lice can slow down their systems for a long time, much the way humans slow down their systems when they get hypothermia, as a survival mechanism. So it takes a long time for the lice to actually die.

After the oil has been in the hair for six to eight hours, comb out the still-oily hair with a regular clean comb to remove tangles. Then use a good metal nit comb to remove both nits and lice.

Proper combing is a crucial step in eliminat-

Heads Up

If you wash out the olive oil without combing out the lice first, any lice that are not completely dead will resume activity. So the combing is even more essential to remove adult lice than eggs.

ing head lice. The important thing to remember is that you are combing not just to remove nits *but also to remove persistent nymphs and adults*. This requires two different combing techniques. Both should be done with the olive oil in the hair because some lice may be slowed down or paralyzed but not yet dead. Once the oil is washed off, the lice may revive and be more difficult to comb out. The point here is to *get the lice off the head before you wash out the oil.*

Olive oil also seems to loosen nits, making them easier to comb out—but only while the oil remains on the head.

Combing Technique

Combing to remove bugs: Comb along the entire scalp, with the comb in constant contact with, but not scraping, the scalp. Clean the comb frequently with a tissue.

Don't panic if you comb out a live louse

Head's Up

Olive oil must remain in the hair when combing for lice and nits.

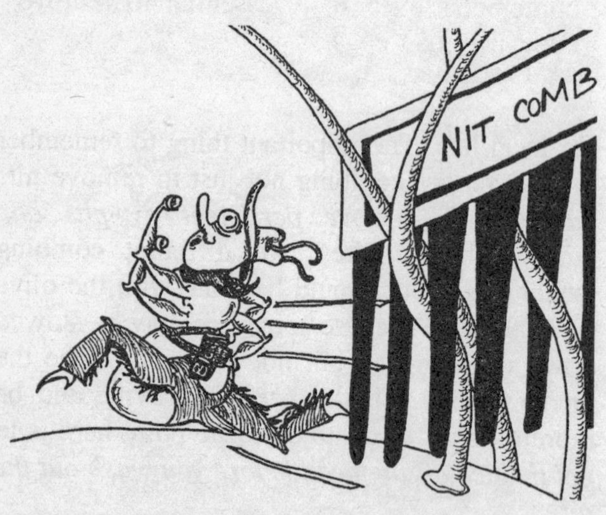

or two. This does not mean that the oil doesn't work. It just means that particular louse didn't get covered sufficiently with the oil, or perhaps it was molting while you were oiling. (Nymphs or baby lice shed their outer shell three times while they are maturing. This interferes with the smothering technique and is why you must continue oiling at specific intervals over the entire three-week cycle.) The fact that the louse is now off your

Nit Comb Review

No one particular louse comb is best for all types of hair and no comb alone will remove all the nits, no matter what the package says or how much you pay for it.

On the other hand, you cannot effectively pick nits without combing because combing is the best way to remove live lice from the head and, until all the lice are removed, they will continue laying eggs and you will be shoveling during a snowstorm.

So, in addition to combing, manual nit removal (picking the nits out with your fingernails) must be a part of every louse treatment program.

The Acumed Lice Comb

This blue metal comb is inexpensive and effective. As it is all metal, it is easy to boil. But people complain that it tears the hair. Best for short or fine hair. Available at most drugstores or from Sawyer Mac Productions at 888-DIE-LICE.

The Licemeister Comb

Shaped like a pick, this comb has long teeth. Many people find it effective in removing nits, especially from very thick or long hair. However, the small handle can cause muscle cramping when used for long periods, and it does not keep hands away from oil. Available only from the National Pediculosis Association, it is expensive.

The Nit Grabber

This newly designed comb has the same graduated long teeth as the Licemeister comb and a long handle to keep hands out of the oil. It has removable teeth and the option of a second set of teeth with shorter prongs. To Order, Call 1-888-DIE-LICE.

child's head is the important part. A louse that is not at least partially covered in oil will easily avoid the nit comb.

Combing to remove nits: Pin hair into sections. Using your fingers, take a very thin section of hair. Starting right at the scalp, comb from the scalp all the way to the end of the hair, being careful not to scrape the scalp. Comb each section several times from different directions and clean the comb frequently with a tissue.

Some people insist, "Oh, I don't need to comb. I can just pick out the nits. It's easier." That's fine for the nits. But until you have combed out live lice, they will continue to lay eggs. You need to get them off the head.

You absolutely must go on to the next step

Nit Comb Testing

Most scientific testing for head lice is actually done on body lice because it is extremely difficult to maintain a colony of head lice in a laboratory. Head lice cannot live on anything other than human blood. Historically, scientists would feed head lice colonies off their own blood, but these days it is more common for scientists to conduct their head lice experiments on body lice. While body lice are similar to head lice in many ways, they can feed off rabbit blood as well as human.

It is important to understand this when you purchase a nit comb that claims to have tested "100% effective." Body lice eggs are slightly larger than head lice eggs. Also the female head louse secures her egg more firmly to a hair shaft than the female body louse secures her egg to a fabric fiber. Therefore, while a given nit comb may indeed be 100% effective in removing body lice eggs in a laboratory, it probably won't be 100% effective in removing head lice eggs from a person's scalp.

This doesn't mean that it isn't a good nit comb. It does mean that it is vital to go through the scalp and manually remove any eggs that the comb missed. Nor does this mean that it is OK to skip the combing and simply remove all the eggs manually. As we've said before, you must comb to remove live lice as well as nits. And you cannot remove the live lice unless they are combed out while their systems are shut down by olive oil.

and pick out any nits you've missed. But before that you must wash out the oil.

Hair-Washing Technique

For the first wash, pour plenty of clarifying shampoo for oily hair directly onto the oily head. Don't wet the head until you have worked the shampoo through the hair. *Then rinse* and lather again. Olive oil is fairly easy to remove. Two to three lathers should do the trick. We have found that Clairol Herbal Essence Clarifying Shampoo for Oily Hair works well, but most clarifying shampoos will do the job.

Remember, *lice are killed by dry heat*. So, dry the hair with a hair dryer, being extremely careful not to burn your child. Children have extremely sensitive scalps.

If your child complains, adjust what you are doing to accommodate your child's comfort level. If your child is comfortable, she will be more willing to cooperate, and everything will go much more quickly and smoothly. Don't forget, you will be repeating this procedure six times over the next three weeks. So make it pleasant and fun or you will be expending precious time and energy chasing the kids down before you even begin.

When the hair is clean and dry it is time to move on to step 5.

STEP 5. CHECK FOR AND REMOVE ANY REMAINING NITS

After the hair has been washed and dried, you must recheck the hair and manually remove any nits that were missed in the combing.

Some organizations that publish louse literature recommend snipping out the hair with the nit attached, using a safety scissors. We find that this process leaves a short hair that can easily end up with another nit on it (since new nits are usually laid right against the scalp) and very short hairs are harder to denit.

We don't recommend that you pull out the hair (a nifty solution suggested by a male entomologist who confessed that he had never actually tried this on a real child). As you probably know, most children will simply not sit still for this. Again, we find that you get much better cooperation if you simply grasp the nit with your fingernail and pull the nit all the way off the hair. Deposit the nit onto an oily tissue, and when you're finished, flush the tissue. (Another male entomologist suggests combing the hair toward the scalp, like teasing, in order to "break the cement holding the nit in place." While this sounds good in theory, we somehow doubt he has tried this on an actual child either.)

Nit removal takes time, but it's a great opportunity to really talk to your child. After all, how often do you get this kind of concentrated time together? If you find you've run out of subjects to talk about, or if you're tense, try a book on tape from a library or bookstore. Books on tape are superior to videos because with videos, the child wants to look up at the TV when you need his or her head down.

Books on tape are a great way to experience the classics (or any book) together. Joan's whole family got addicted to books on tape while we were nit-picking.

If your child is tired, let her sit at a counter and rest her head on her arms. Many children sleep through long hours of nit-picking this way.

When you have finished removing the nits, be sure to wash your hands carefully and use a nailbrush. Lice like to hide under nails.

If you have a badly infested child with waist-length hair, you have a decision to make. Is it worth cutting the child's hair?

That's for you and your child to decide together. There is absolutely no reason to cut hair any shorter than shoulder length unless the child specifically wants short hair. However, getting nits out of waist-length hair can be tedious and increases the chances of losing a nit in the hair. So, you and your child should make this decision together.

The problem is that no matter how careful you are, you probably will miss a few nits—everyone does. Many experienced school nurses and parents swear that nits are getting smaller over time. This would make sense, due to natural selection because the smallest nits would be more difficult to spot and eliminate, and therefore more likely to survive. But to our knowledge, no one has studied this phenomenon.

So, repeat treatments are timed to catch any louse that hatches from an unpicked nit, after it hatches and before it's old enough to lay eggs of it's own. Since it takes eight to ten days for a nymph (baby louse) to mature, we have found the following treatment procedure to be the most effective with every infestation:

Repeat Steps 2 (the olive oil), 4 (the comb-out), and 5 (the nit check) on the following days over the three-week life cycle of the louse. Days 1, 5, 9, 13, 17, and 21. Add Day 2 if you chose not to use a pediculicide.

This protocol has been tested extensively by us on many lousy families and it has worked

The Nit-Picking Technique

Divide the hair and pull one-half of the hair into a ponytail. Check the other side by systematically moving around the head and pinning the hair out of the way as you finish each strand.

Take a thin strand of hair in your fingers and check both sides of the hair carefully for nits. Remember, the newest nits are smallest and closest to the scalp. These are the most difficult to see. If your eyes aren't great, we recommend using a vision visor—a binocular magnifier that fits over your head like goggles, leaving both hands free. It magnifies two and a half times at eight inches and helps to find those nits. You can also use a magnifying lamp, but these can be expensive.

This is a critical time. The harder you work now, the easier it will be later. It is important to remove every single nit for several reasons:

1) So the nit won't hatch and lay more eggs.
2) So you know if there are any live lice left on the head that are laying new nits.
3) So if your school has a no-nit policy (see Chapter 5), your child can return to school.

every time, when it is done correctly.

Now, before you decide that this is too much work, think about how much cleaning, combing, and picking you did on that first day. Don't trip at the finish line. Too many folks get cocky and are convinced they've gotten every nit and louse and they can skip the last couple of treatments because it's not convenient. They're the ones who end up leaving work early three weeks later to pick up their kids and start the whole process all over again.

5

School, Day Care, and Community Management of Head Lice

There is no other health condition which seems to create greater chaos in the school system than does head lice. . . .

—Janis Hootman, RN, Ph.D., CSN (Certified School Nurse), and head of research for the National Association of School Nurses in the American Academy of Pediatric News

Every parent with an elementary-age child is familiar with the dreaded notice that begins "A child in your son/daughter's class has head lice. Please check your child." The notice usually goes on to explain what head lice and nits look like and then outlines a basic program for eliminating them. The program typically suggests that parents use a pediculicide, clean the house, and check and remove nits. Reasonable, but in

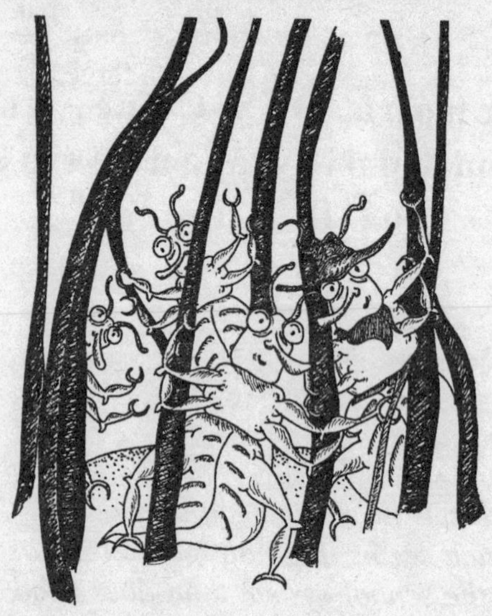

Eight out of ten school districts in the United States reported at least one case of head lice in 1998.

the age of persistent head lice infestations, an inadequate response. These days schools should play a more active role than just sending notices home.

Most often, in school settings the management of head lice is placed squarely in the lap of the school nurse. But these days, to be effective, pediculosis management requires a broader approach. While the school nurse is the logical person to be in charge of school head lice management, she should be part of a larger head lice management team.

Everyone needs to be prepared and accountable for his or her part of the program, and each of these groups has a vital role to play in making sure that a head-louse problem on one child does not spread throughout the class or school. When everyone is properly educated *before* a crisis, head-louse infestations can be brought under control quickly and efficiently.

Head-louse infestations cause so much stress for families and schools that an appropriate head-louse management program should be a high priority for any school. Every school head lice management team should be responsible for designing a set of guidelines for head-louse management for their community. Those guidelines should be distributed at the start of each school year to principals, teachers, guidance counselors, librarians, parents, the Parent Teacher Organization and the local newspaper.

THE PARENTS' ROLE

Parents need to step up to the plate and do what it takes to get rid of a head-louse infestation on their child. They cannot expect the school nurse to be in charge of the home treatment plan or to act as resident nit-picker for their child. School nurses simply do not have the time.

Heads Up

Head lice management teams should include school nurses, teachers, parents, counselors, and school administrators.

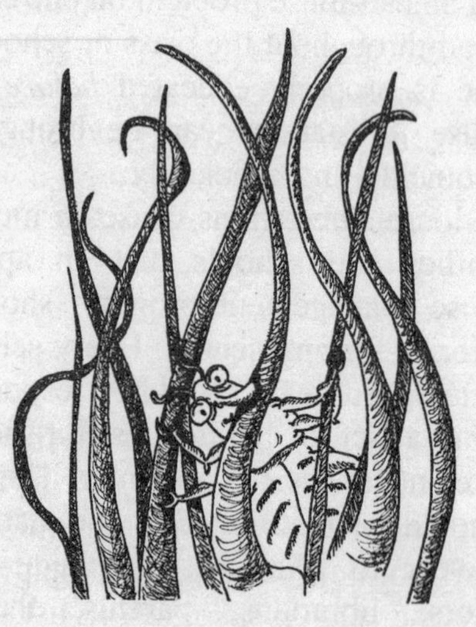

The good news is that all parents can do the job as long as they have been armed with the right information and are diligent in following an integrated treatment protocol, like the Five-Step Battle Plan. If parents receive complete, up-to-date information about how to treat head lice from their school nurse and are encouraged to follow through with a multistep treatment program, the chances are excellent that the infestation will be controlled and an epidemic will be avoided.

If you are a working parent, or have several children and need help with nit removal, check with your local public health department to see if they know anyone who will come to your home to help you. If the health department can't or won't help, try the local Visiting Nurses Association. Some health departments and nurses' associations are more helpful than others. Also, ask around town to see if anyone knows about professional nit-picking services, or check with the American Head Lice Information Center for a list of resources in your area. (See Resource list in the back of this book.) If all of these options fail, ask a friend or a family member to help you. Offer to help in return if the situation is reversed in the future, or barter some babysitting. If you can afford it, you could offer to pay the school nurse to come and help you after school. Some schools also keep a list of people willing to help others through an infestation.

If you are the parent of a school-age child, stay informed about head lice. The better prepared you are, the less likely you are to panic. Keep some bandannas, shower caps, olive oil, and a few nit combs in your linen closet. That way you won't have to run to the drugstore in the middle of the night when you discover lice on your child.

The following guidelines will help prevent

head lice from becoming a major annoyance for everyone in the school community.

THE SCHOOL'S RESPONSIBILITIES

The key to controlling head lice is education. Therefore, every school should develop an information package for distribution to parents and teachers. The package should be updated every year and passed out at the start of each school year to every parent and teacher. Extra copies should be available on request.

The following items should be included in the information package:

- Basic information on identifying head lice.
- An alert that pediculicides may no longer be 100 percent effective.
- A warning against overusing pediculicides.
- A clear outline of school policies, such as the no-nit policy discussed later in this chapter.
- Complete instructions on how to eliminate head lice safely.
- A list of which treatments to avoid.
- Emphasis on the importance of regular head-louse checks by the parent.
- School pickup and return policies for an infested child.
- An introduction to the olive oil treatment protocol.

This information package should also be distributed to the school and town library systems. Each library system should have a section on head lice, which includes books, videos, articles, and a display of lice removal products. Somc schools and Parent-Teacher Organizations have worked together and designed creative displays for back-to-school nights.

THE TEACHERS' ROLE

Teachers should be trained to recognize signs of head lice, such as excessive scratching, irritability, or the presence of nits and/or lice. Teachers should be given proper guidelines on how to send the child to the school nurse without embarrassing or stigmatizing him or her. They should treat head lice as a part of everyday life, just like colds, flu, or chicken pox.

If it is confirmed that a child has lice, the school nurse should thoroughly check every child in the classroom and any siblings in the school. If a sibling attends a different school, the school nurse there should be alerted.

Teachers should supervise the separation of coats and hats to prevent the further spread of head lice. Kids can tuck their hats and scarves into their coat sleeves. Some schools mandate that children bring laundry bags to store their coats in during an outbreak.

Teachers should distribute louse alert notices to all homes.

If the head louse management team has done its job, parents will have enough information to handle the problem without panicking.

THE CHILD'S ROLE

School-age children can be an important part of a head louse management program. At the beginning of each school year, the school nurse or a trained volunteer should go around to each classroom and educate children about head lice. Children should be taught the symptoms of head lice, what head lice and their nits look like, how head lice spread, and what they themselves can do to minimize their chances of getting head lice. Many schools use the humorous video *Head Lice to Dead Lice* to teach this information.

Both teachers and children should be made aware that having head lice is not a sin but a health problem comparable to a head cold and that teasing about head lice is unkind and unacceptable. Fear of teasing may prevent children from reporting symptoms of an infestation, which could lead to more widespread contamination. All children should be encouraged to tell their parents, teacher, or school nurse any time their head itches. A child should be confident enough to request a head check at any time without fear of embarrassment.

Schools can help with diagnosis by implementing regular louse checks. Children frequently return to school from vacations and camps having been exposed to new people and their head lice. Schools should be ready with a trained team of parents or nurses to check every head in the school after major vacations—summer, Thanksgiving, Christmas, winter and spring breaks. Working these checks into the overall school schedule is one of the best ways to keep head lice from spreading throughout a classroom, school, and community. Checks can be done right in the classroom to minimize disruption. Teasing is less likely to be a problem if children are properly prepared with information about head lice ahead of time.

Because it is relatively easy to misdiagnose head lice, people who know what they are looking for should perform head checks. The school nurse should conduct a training session at the beginning of every school year for volunteers. Volunteers should see an actual louse and nit, be shown how to use lice sticks (like small popsicle sticks used by school nurses to probe the scalp during a lice check) to separate the hair, and where and how to check the head for nits and lice. The video *Head Lice to Dead Lice,* which includes a proper nit check demonstration as well as basic information on head lice, can be a helpful training aid.

When a child is identified as having head lice, everyone else in that class, including the teacher, should be checked weekly for a month. Parents should be notified and made aware that they need to check their children daily for a month to make sure that they don't develop signs of an infestation. It is a good idea for everyone in the class to do one olive-oil treatment (see Chapter 4 for directions) and a comb-out. This will get rid of adult lice and buy everyone time to continue checking for nits. As the nits get older, they grow larger and move farther from the scalp so they can be seen more easily. At this stage, an infestation is more obvious to people with less experience.

During an Outbreak

- Check the heads of everyone in the class and have parents check siblings. Parents should check each other's heads as well.
- Check everyone who has been exposed, weekly for four weeks.
- Monitor infested students carefully for four weeks.
- If parents are having a hard time controlling an infestation, demonstrate a proper nit check and make sure they know what they are looking for and are capable of spotting lice and nits.

- Make sure parents have an up-to-date information package and suggest that they try the olive oil protocol.
- Recommend that students with long hair come to school with their hair in braids.
- Hang coats and hats in separate cubbies or in bags.
- Make sure that children do not share brushes, headgear, pillows, or bedding.
- Visually inspect and clean athletic headgear and life vests between uses.

PROPER CLEANING OF THE SCHOOL ENVIRONMENT

When a school or a classroom experiences an outbreak of head lice, follow these cleaning procedures:

- All classrooms with carpets should be vacuumed thoroughly daily.
- All headgear should be wiped down with the school's regular cleaning solutions or vacuumed.
- Louse sprays are not recommended. The Centers for Disease Control is against their use because they are dangerous to small children and pets. Also, they may be ineffective due to resistance.
- Coats and hats should not touch each other. If hooks are too close together, or if indi-

vidual cubbies are unavailable, individual laundry bags with drawstrings can be used to store coats and hats.

- It's best to curtail dress-up play completely during an outbreak. If this isn't possible, dress-up clothes should be put in a hot dryer every evening for twenty minutes.
- Day care centers should require parents to take home their child's bedding every night for laundering and drying.
- Bedding should not be shared, particularly during an outbreak.
- Be especially aware of head-lice management when sharing costumes for a school play. Costumes should not be shared or rotated without being cleaned between uses.

These precautions will help any facility control an outbreak.

SHOULD YOUR SCHOOL HAVE A NO-NIT POLICY?

The No-Nit Policy is a somewhat controversial policy recommended by the National Pediculosis Association. This policy calls for the "exclusion of a child from a school setting, camp or day care facility until the child is completely free of lice, nits, and egg cases (empty louse eggs)." It also recommends community education so that parents understand their responsibilities under this policy, which many schools have implemented to control widespread lice infestations.

Advantages of a No-Nit Policy

- It forces parents to remove all the nits. When you have achieved ground zero, and new nits appear, it means there are still live lice on the head and that further action (preferably the smothering technique) is necessary.
- Parents and schools will know when a child has been nit free for ten days and the infestation is over.

Disadvantages of a No-Nit Policy

- No-nit policies can be carried out too rigidly. Some children, whose parents are doing their best to control resistant infestations but are armed with insufficient information, can be kept our of school for days, weeks, and months. In some cases, children have been removed from their parents' custody by well-meaning but overly rigid social service agencies because they have missed too much school due to head lice. This should not occur.
- Head lice can be misdiagnosed easily. According to Dr. Richard Pollack of the Harvard School of Public Health, many of the

samples of "head lice" sent to him from parents and school nurses do not turn out to be head lice but various hair debris, dandruff, or DEC (desquamated epithelial cell) plugs, which are caused by overusing pediculicides or hair sprays. If a child with DEC plugs is being misdiagnosed and is constantly sent home for treatment, it will cause endless frustration for families and schools, and overtreatment can be a hazard to a child. Before a school sends a child home, specimens should be checked under a microscope to ensure a correct diagnosis. It's easy to spot nits under a microscope. They have a distinctive cap on the end. When a nit has hatched, the cap is no longer intact.

We recommend that a no-nit policy be openly discussed with parents, teachers, and the school nurse. Use the policy as a guideline and allow the nurse leeway in administering it. No child should be forced out of school for long periods because of head lice. If a child is sent home more than twice, the information being supplied to the family is not adequate, or the family is having difficulty doing the nit checks. Get the family some help.

Dr. Pollack also favors a moderate approach. On his web page on head lice, he states: "Common sense, clear guidelines, and a dose of humanity should be the rules of thumb when schools are dealing with head lice."

Because proper diagnosis is often not ensured, these policies are often misapplied. Children should not lose time from school, parents should not lose time from work, and treatment is not indicated if the infestation is not active. Lice on children's heads, by themselves, should not be cause for the schools or courts to label the parents as "neglectful." Such extreme reactions to an infestation are generally unwarranted and may suggest poor judgment on the part of those making policy decisions.

What to Avoid

- School nurses should not apply pediculicides to children's heads or require them to be used. The decision to use a pediculicide should be made by informed parents. Pediculicides should not be used on any child under six months of age and preferably not on anyone under three years of age. They should also never be used on women who are pregnant or nursing, or anyone with cuts or abrasions on the head. Check the packaging for other restrictions.

- Schools do not need to hire specialized firms to disinfect the school during a head-louse outbreak. Cleaning the school is important, but complicated methods and special cleaning supplies are unnecessary.
- Never stigmatize a child with head lice.

The following is a sample school notice to parents informing them that a child in their child's class has head lice. The letter should include a photograph or a drawing of lice and nits. It is also helpful to show their actual sizes.

Dear Parent or Guardian:

Someone in your child's class has been diagnosed with head lice. We have already performed a head check on your child and did not find any signs of head lice. However, please continue to check your child's head and scalp for signs of head lice or nits (lice eggs) for a month. Head lice are contagious, so check siblings and any adults living in the house. Pets do not get head lice.

If you find signs of lice, don't panic. The information package we are sending will tell you everything you need to know about eliminating head lice.

If you decide to use a pediculicide

(louse-killing shampoo or creme rinse), please check with your pharmacist or physician and choose the correct product for each family member. Follow the directions on the package and do not overuse the treatments.

Because some populations of head lice have developed resistance to some pesticides, pediculicides may no longer be fully effective in eliminating head lice. Therefore, you may need to take additional steps to make sure the infestation is completely cleared. Recommended steps include: regular nit checks and manual nit-picking over the 21-day life cycle of the louse, the olive oil protocol and the P-V-P housecleaning method outlined in the book and video entitled *Head Lice to Dead Lice* or the cleaning methods outlined in *The Lice Buster Book.* Copies of these books are available in the school library.

Your child will be allowed to return to school when the school nurse has determined that the infestation is under control and is no longer contagious.

Head lice are a normal part of school life. Head lice prefer clean healthy heads, and the presence of head lice is not a reflection of poor hygiene. Please remember that head lice do not spread illness, nor are they life threatening. If you need additional help or advice, please contact one of the following volunteers:

(List names and phone numbers of people willing to help.)

6 Prevention: Keep Those Creatures Away

Once you've been through a louse infestation, you never want to go through it again. No one does. It's simply too much work. The best news is that there's a good chance you won't have to because you and your family know a lot more now about what causes an infestation and will automatically behave differently knowing what you now know.

Here are some pointers to help avoid future infestations:

- *Show your kids the video Head Lice to Dead Lice: Safe Solutions for Frantic Families* (or any other video/educational material). It is very funny. Comedian Paul Wagner plays the mother, father, and school nurse. He is also the voice of an animated louse, Nit Pickens. Kids love this video and therefore will watch it over and

People cannot get head lice from pets and pets cannot get head lice from people.

over. And by watching it again and again, they soak up the information and make it a part of their everyday lives. It's amazing how easily and conscientiously kids will avoid behaviors that expose them to head lice when they understand head lice and how people catch them. At the end of the video, kids give the rules for avoiding an infestation (see sidebar). And when kids have heard these rules enough times, they become a sort of mantra, ingrained into their subconscious.

- *When you go to see a children's movie in a theater*, take along a rain slicker and throw it over the back of the seat. This way your child won't put his head back against a seat that has just held an infested child. When you leave, shake out the slicker. Lice can't cling to slick material.
- *When you fly or take a train or bus*, either don't put your head back or take a quick look at the seat back before you do. Lice aren't invisible. If there is a louse, you will see it. Or, if you are seriously traumatized by your head-louse experience, take along a lint remover and go over the back of the

Rules for Kids

Wear your hair up.

You can share candy but you can't share hats.

Keep your brushes and combs to yourself.

Follow the Battle Plan.

If you get head lice, don't panic, they can't hurt you.

Tell your mom to check your head every week.

Anyone can get head lice.

Remember, if your friend gets head lice, don't make fun of him or her because you might be next.

seat. It will make you feel better. Just be prepared to share your lint remover with others on the plane.

- *If there is a head-louse epidemic in your area*, go over your car seats with a lint remover after driving car pool.
- *When your child returns from summer camp*, use olive oil the night she returns home, whether you see signs of lice or not. Then put everything possible through a hot dryer for at least twenty minutes. Thoroughly clean combs and brushes. Remember all that hugging and kissing that went

on the last day of camp? Check her head that night and then a week later.

- *Any time you hear about an infestation in your child's classroom*, you can use olive oil, comb out the hair the next morning, wash and dry the hair, and then check for nits. Check again in a week, and use the olive oil again if you wish. As long as your child is not allergic to olives (if she is, choose another food-based oil), the olive oil won't hurt and it is great for the hair. If a couple of lice have gotten on the child's head, you will get them off quickly. Once you have eliminated the live lice, you have a few days to remove the nits.
- *During an outbreak of head lice, it is important for children to keep their hair to themselves and close to their heads.* The less swing and sway at this time, the better. French braids are the best possible hairstyle for girls. We have also found that "the wet look" appears to act as a deterrent for head lice because the female has a hard time cementing the nits to oily hair. Therefore, a little coconut or olive oil left on the hair during a school outbreak won't hurt and may help, as long as the child doesn't mind.
- *If you must try on hats in a store*, look at the insides before you or your child put them on your head.

- *If you buy clothes at a used clothing establishment or if you take clothing out of the lost and found,* wash them then dry them in a hot dryer if possible.
- *Become active in establishing head-lice policies in your school.* Make sure your school nurse has information on how and why olive oil works. Try to educate parents ahead of time so they don't depend on false or outdated information. Remember, it is in your best interest to help other parents get rid of an infestation quickly.
- *Volunteer to help your school nurse* with regular head checks now that you're an expert at spotting nits.
- *Encourage your school nurse to schedule regular head checks* after all major school vacations. Help with the nit checks or raise money to hire someone who knows what to look for.
- *Support your school nurse.* And don't play the blame game.
- *Start a fund at school to help parents* who can't afford olive oil and metal nit combs. You'll end up saving money and time in the long run by not catching other people's lice.
- *Organize a nit-picking posse* to help mothers learn how to check their children, help parents who are visually challenged, and

check the heads of parents who need extra help.

- *Stand firm* with the school nurse about implementing a no-nits policy in your school. However, make sure this policy is used with intelligent discretion. There is no need to send a child home with two nits if the family is using the olive oil correctly and consistently, or if the school nurse believes that the family has the problem under control. But you may encounter people who refuse to take the time to get rid of all the nits. This is where the power of a no-nits policy can help. It will force the parent to spend the time to get rid of all the nits. Interestingly enough, some people who have the most difficulty spending the necessary time are families where both parents are busy professionals.
- *Make head checks a pleasant experience* for the children. If you cause your child stress over lice, he will hesitate to come to you if his head itches. From a child's point of view, head lice aren't so bad. He gets to miss a couple of days of school and gets lots of extra time with Mom or Dad. And many people love the feeling of having their heads checked. During the head checks, listen to a book on tape. (Don't play a video, as the child won't want to

keep his head down or turned to the side when you need him to.)

If worse comes to worse and you do get lice again, you will recognize it much earlier.

- You will check your child the minute you see him scratch that special scratch.
- You will know what to look for. You will recognize those tiny oval eggs attached at an angle to the hair shaft.
- You will have all your tools on hand, including a large bottle of cheap olive oil, a shower cap, and a metal nit comb suited to your child's hair. Your child will be less likely to object to combing if the nit comb you have on hand doesn't pull or rip the hair.
- If you see your child scratching late at night, you will have what you need to apply the olive oil, comb out the hair in the morning, and check the olive oil for lice as you comb to help diagnose an infestation. Then take a long leisurely look for nits when you and your child are not so tired. It can even wait until your child comes home from school, because the oil will eliminate the adult lice that can migrate to another child.
- Tell the school nurse and the parents of your friends immediately if your family is

infested. Help your friends catch it early. That way they'll be less likely to pass it back to you or your children.

- If your child or your child's friend has head lice, don't have sleepovers for the three weeks the child is being treated for lice. If sleepovers cannot be avoided, have everyone at the sleepover do the olive oil treatment that night to prevent contagion. For girls you can think of it as a great night of beauty and do everyone's nails while you're at it.

Here are some other general pointers:

- Children get other creatures in their hair besides lice, especially when they play outside. Many times a renegade aphid in the hair will cause a mother to panic. If it flies away, it is not a louse. Lice don't have wings.
- If your child has suspicious bites other than on the head, check your bedding for body lice, bedbugs, mites, or fleas. Bedbugs are much larger than lice and are dark red in color; mites are much smaller than lice and are also often red in color. Should these be found, contact the school nurse. Even though body lice are unusual except on the homeless, sometimes you don't know who slept on a mattress before you or your

child. Body lice lay their eggs in the seams of clothes and mattresses. If you see lice in bedding, get rid of the bedding or dry what you can in a hot dryer. Replace the mattress if you possibly can or vacuum it thoroughly. Then make sure all clothes are dried in a hot dryer.

- If you have used a pediculicide that didn't work, take it back to the pharmacy and get your money back. If the pharmacy won't help you, send it back to the manufacturer for a refund. Warner Lambert has promised to return the cost of Nix as part of a settlement of a threatened class action suit. Readers should spread the word about ineffective pediculicides.

When you have conscientiously completed your three weeks of lice and nit removal, it's time to get on with your lives. Don't freak out every time your head itches or you see your child scratch his head. Many women who have had a traumatic experience with head lice are sure they still have it months after the last louse has been obliterated. It is very common for women to have a visceral reaction to their heads itching after surviving a head-lice infestation, much like posttraumatic stress disorder. It's as if an alarm goes off in their heads screaming: "*Danger, danger, nest has been invaded.*"

Just because you itch doesn't mean you have

head lice. Lots of things can make you itch, like allergies, or dry, overtreated scalps, or lint. If you're worried, have someone you trust take a look or use olive oil to diagnose the problem. When you use your nit comb to comb out the oil, take a look at what comes out. If it doesn't have legs, it's not a louse.

Now take a deep breath and a nice hot bath. You've earned it. And give yourself a great big A in Head Lice 101.

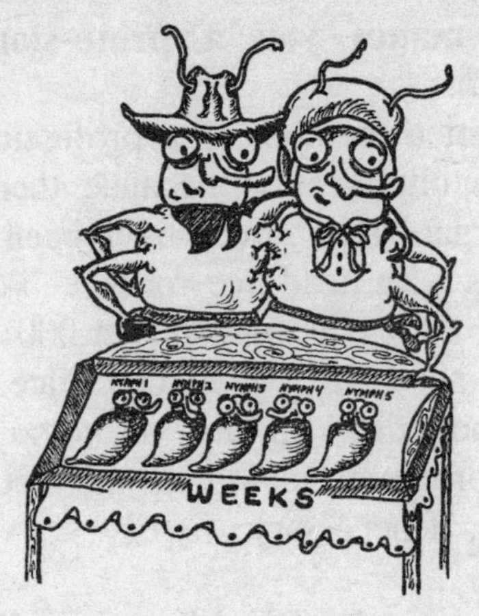

7
Confessions of a Professional Nit-Picker

Mary Ward is a professional nit-picker residing in Cambridge, Massachusetts. She is featured in the December 1998 issue of *National Geographic.*

What makes you a professional nit-picker?
I am not a member of a professional nit-picking organization because there is no such organization, but I have been helping families with head lice for three years and I work with approximately 1,000 infested people per year. Many desperate parents and schools call and ask me to solve their louse problem, including the actual nit-picking, if necessary.

How do you begin with a new client?
I ask new clients to describe the history of their infestation and what they have tried so far, and then I give advice. If they need it, I will come and help remove nits, or show them how to do it.

Sometimes I find out that it's not lice and they've been treating for lice. But the majority of people who come to me do have lice and have been trying unsuccessfully to kill them with chemicals. Then they run into school systems or physicians that blame the family instead of the chemical for being unsuccessful.

What is your opinion about using pediculicides to treat head lice?
From my observations, chemicals are not doing a great job in controlling head lice

right now, at least in the Boston area. And there are countless media reports about other parts of the country having chronic lice problems as well, so I think the problem is pretty widespread.

My advice regarding chemicals is that if a product doesn't work the first time, it's not likely to work the second, third, or fourth time. If you used the product the way you are supposed to, and there are still live lice, the product didn't work. So, don't use it anymore. Accept the fact that you are going to have to try another method to get rid of the infestation.

Please understand that I am not anti-chemical. I just don't believe in subjecting children to chemical products that are not working. It doesn't make sense.

And I tell the client that I don't know of any chemicals, even prescription medications that are currently safe and reliable in getting rid of louse problems. If it's a very early case, some people may get rid of lice using the chemicals, but most people are going to need something more.

What methods do you recommend for getting rid of head lice?

I usually recommend a smothering technique using olive oil because it is safe and mostly nonallergenic, so it can be used over and over again without any side effects. However, it's difficult to smother a head louse on a head. It's not difficult to smother them with oil in a laboratory, but a head is not a petri dish.

Most people I speak to are willing to try the olive oil procedure. Some don't want to try it because it seems like so much more time on top of the time that they've already spent. But those people who resist usually call me back the next week, because they still have head lice and now they are ready to try smothering them.

I won't work with people who won't smother the lice because it's a waste of their money and my time.

I explain that I need the whole family to be treated before I get there. They need to cover their hair and scalp completely with olive oil, and leave it on at least six or eight hours.

The most important step is to comb through the hair very carefully before they wash out the oil. They're using a nit comb, but they're combing to get rid of adult lice. Most people will find some dead lice, but the majority of the lice are just slowed down. They're not dead yet. Only a few lice are actually killed with the olive oil, so it's essential to comb out all of those lice while they're slowed down. Once you wash out the oil, remaining lice start moving around just as fast as they did before.

Have you found that olive oil kills all the live lice?

There's a stage in the life cycle of the louse when the bug is not easily killed or slowed down or gotten rid of in any way with the oil. This stage seems to be the newly hatched lice (nymphs) from the first day they're hatched until they're about four days old. I can't explain why that happens; it's just what I see on all people. So it's important to repeat the olive oil treatment on specific days during the three-week period, in order to get each louse at the right stage. I can't stress that enough.

I'm waiting for at least *ten days of no nits* to be sure the infestation is over. Not all people actually need the entire three weeks, because if they have an early case and they get to *ten days nit free* early on, they can stop.

Most people will come up with zero nits, zero nits, and all of a sudden they see four, five, six, eight nits. When they see that jump in the number of nits, they know that they have an adult louse on their head that's laying eggs, and they can try oil that same day to get rid of that adult louse. Oil works very well with adult lice, but the family has to go back to zero in terms of being ten days nit free.

What about nit-picking?

What I tell them is that if they do the oil treatment for three weeks, it usually covers even people who aren't great nit-pickers. But I want them to become great nit-pickers because it's essential to get rid of all the lice eggs. You don't know that you're done with an infestation until all the nits are gone.

As far as I can tell, nothing is killing those eggs. You have to remove them. With some encouragement most people can learn how to look at their child's head enough so that they can be comfortable saying I have no nits. Or I have a few nits. The cop-out—"I can't nit-pick"—is not going to help them get rid of lice.

A lot of people at the beginning will say "I can't see them." But usually they can. They just have to learn what to look for and what not to look for.

What should they look for?

Almost everything that isn't a nit will come off the hair by flicking it off or brushing it off, or you pull it halfway off the hair and it falls off or crumbles between your fingers. A nit does not crumble between your fingers. It has to be pulled off the entire shaft of hair. If you're pulling a nit off and you go halfway off the hair, you can let go of it, and it will still be stuck to that hair. Another helpful hint is that if you can get the nit off the hairshaft using only one finger, it's not a nit. That helps most parents distinguish between things that are nits and things that aren't nits.

What are some problems you encounter with families cooperating?

Sometimes the whole family doesn't want to do the olive oil at the same time. But I tell them that it doesn't help to have one person do the olive oil protocol and not the others. Sometimes it makes it worse, depending on how bad a case they have, because adult lice can be passed from someone who hasn't done the treatment to someone who has.

Everyone in the family needs to do the oil treatment on the same day so that they are all at the same stage at the same time. And you can keep better track of things if everybody's on the same schedule.

What difference do you see between families who use the olive oil and families who don't?

You can get rid of head lice without the olive oil if you remove all the nits and all

I don't know of any comb that can get rid of all the nits on a head.
—Mary Ward

the insects manually. But most of us do not have the skills or the patience to remove every egg and every louse. And we're certainly not able to do that if we're just using a comb.

I know combs that do a very, very good job, and different combs do different jobs for different types of hair.

Sometimes I'll pull thirty lice off of a child's head. But I stress to parents that just because I've pulled off fifteen or thirty does not mean I've controlled the problem. It means there's still a lot of lice that I didn't find, and we still need to try to get rid of them. Oil is a great tool for us. But it's not a quick fix.

Unless you use the olive oil on the right days and in the right way, you won't be successful. Other people try to smother lice different ways. I haven't seen it used successfully unless it is combined with thorough combing, with the smothering agent still on the head, very careful nit-picking, and repeated use of the smothering agent on very specific days. It's not an easy thing to do.

What sort of things do you look for when you go into a home?

When I walk into a home, I glance around to see what the family's doing to control the lice. Usually I see plastic bags all over and vacuum cleaners out because they've been vacuuming like maniacs. This tells me that I have to get them back into focusing on the head, not the environment.

Sometimes I walk into a home and they haven't done anything to control the environment. They have couches that haven't been vacuumed forever. You can see hair all over. I might encourage that family to deal with the environment.

Then they say "Here, hang your coat right here" and I say "No. I don't think so." I tell them not to hang their coats together until the problem is over.

What are some ways that you think people spread head lice?

The most common way to spread head lice is head-to-head contact.

When I see an entire family that all have lice, it's usually because everybody is using the same brush. Lice can spread through that family very quickly. When a family doesn't use the same brush, there are often people who don't have it. I ask them, "Do you use the same brush?" and if they say "Yes," almost always everybody in the family has it.

How do children spread head lice in schools?

Most often kids spread head lice through head-to-head contact. I suspect that coats hung right next to each other in open cubbies are also a way to share head lice because once the head gets overpopulated, the lice are going to crawl off onto the coat. That louse is looking for a new head. It's moving around. It doesn't want to stay on a coat, so it can move to another coat. That doesn't mean that everybody in the class is going to get it because one coat had a louse on it. It may mean that the person whose coat is right next to that coat will get it. You can't all get lice from one louse on one coat.

Usually whole classrooms get it because nobody's looking at the heads. Most often children have complained about their heads being itchy long before an entire class gets checked. When I've seen whole classes infested, it's usually because one or two people a month ago said, "I was really itching and I asked somebody to look at me, and they didn't see anything, or they said I had really bad dandruff." Throughout that month of children doing things together, an entire class could become infested quite easily.

Many entomologists are adamant that you cannot contract head lice through a vector, like a brush or a towel. It has to be head-to-head contact.

Well, I can tell you positively that I've seen live head lice on brushes and combs. In really bad cases, I've seen moving lice in the bathroom, on the floor and on towels.

It used to be that when Richard [Pollack, entomologist at the Harvard School of Public Health] would ask me, "How many lice do you typically see on a head?" I'd say, "Not very many."

These days [1999], I sometimes see thirty or forty on a head. That's more typical now than three or four. Now, do I think you're going to pass it quickly when you have three, four, or even eight lice on a head? No. But I think you can pass it really quickly when you see thirty. That's pretty easy to spread through brushes.

Why are there so many more lice on each head now?

I think there are two reasons. The first one is ignorance and lack of information. The second is that we're being duped. We're told that the chemicals work. We're told this by physicians, school nurses, teachers, and the media all the time. There are lice chemical commercials on TV every single day, more than I've ever seen in my entire life.

The advertisements tell us that these chemicals work 99 percent of the time. So, we go home, we treat our children, and we send them back to school, sometimes with almost the same number of lice that they left school the day before with. But we come back to school with a false sense of security. We think we have gotten rid of the problem. We're trying to kill head lice with chemicals and we're not killing them. So, the lice are multiplying, and we're seeing more because we're sending the children back so they can infest more children. Nobody's making sure that those children are clear.

I'm not against a school telling people to use chemicals. But schools have to follow through to make sure that those children are done with lice. And often schools will find that if they really follow through, those children aren't done with lice. They're not even close to being done. Then, all of a sudden, more children in the classroom have lice. How did that happen? Well, it happens because those first few children didn't get rid of the lice.

There are more lice, not because all of a sudden lice are superlice that multiply twice as fast. It's that parents and schools are not taking care of the problem. We don't check our children's heads, and when we do, we don't know what to look for. Most parents say "Well, she really itched, and I looked, but quite honestly, I didn't know what I was looking for."

If you're going to be handing out advice, you'd better follow through to make sure that your advice is good. Often the school nurse says, "I want you to treat with Nix or Rid." So, the children go home, and the nurse checks them the next day and says, "Well, you still have a few nits, but don't worry, there are no lice." You can't assume there are no lice just because you used a pesticide and the company says it's 99 percent effective. You can't see the lice that are left because they hide from the light.

Unless the school and the parents follow through to make sure that the children are done, the heads will get saturated with bugs and lice will eventually spread throughout the school.

What do you recommend for schools?

I recommend that schools become educated. Chemicals are hardly ever a quick fix anymore. Sometimes they work, but right now, in many areas, they're not doing the trick. Once the school understands that, they can deal with the problem a lot better.

Schools can consider other options, like mechanically removing nits and mechanically killing lice. Smothering is a way to kill lice mechanically. People come to schools for good advice. "What am I supposed to do about this? I've never seen it before. You're a school. You've seen it before. What do I do?"

I think it's very important for all the teachers, not just administrators or nurses, to understand what lice and nits look like, because parents will ask teachers directly. So, you need teachers to be willing and able to help in that process.

It's essential to try and limit the number of lice cases per year, and the only way to limit that number is to identify cases of head lice as quickly as possible. Schools need very thorough lice checks, not spot checks where they take a Popsicle stick and look right behind the ear and at the nape of the neck. Spot checks will probably not identify new cases.

You want to be able to identify a head-louse infestation when it's a week old, not three weeks old. And, don't just look for lice. Look for evidence on the head. If there are bites, investigate further. Check again in a couple of days if you see bites on the head, even if you don't see nits.

How long should nit checks take?

When I'm in a school, I'll take forty-five minutes or an hour in a classroom for an entire class, including teachers. That is a good thorough check.

I think schools need to set up regular head-check programs at specific times of the year, like the beginning of school and after certain breaks, like Thanksgiving. But also it's a good idea for the teacher to check each one of the children once a month during the day. Just look at their heads. Even if the teacher is not perfect at checking for nits, they can identify something suspicious and have a nurse look more carefully. That would keep the number of infestations down a lot.

And once you have cases of lice, monitor them carefully. I'm supportive of the no-nit policy. When a child keeps coming to school with nits, the only way to force the parent to do the best job they can is to send that child home. But if a school nurse knows that the parents are doing everything they can to contain the problem and the child comes with one nit or two nits, I don't necessarily think that child should be sent home. But, in general, the no-nit policy helps contain the problem at school.

But if schools find that they're sending a child home for two weeks or a month, the school is not doing their job. They're not giving that parent enough advice and help to control the problem.

What's the best way to tell a child that he/she has head lice?

If you tell a child very calmly that they have lice, they don't think of it as any more of a problem than if they had mosquito bites or a tick on their head. But if a teacher says "Oh, gross" and tries to keep that child away from everybody as if they're contaminated, it disturbs the child. Anybody can get lice, so it's not like the child did something wrong.

If the child goes home and the mother freaks out, and says it's the worst thing that ever happened in her life, the child will become stressed out. No child will want to sit there and be nit-picked by a parent who's freaking out at him. No way. If every time a mother finds a nit she goes "Oh, damn, I found another nit," that child is not going to sit quietly because he will feel like he did something wrong.

I've found that almost every child with lice knew they had them. They were itchy.

If a child doesn't feel that they can go to someone and say "Please check my head for lice," the child's not going to tell anyone when they itch.

I always say "If you feel itchy again, go tell your teacher or a grown-up to check your head." It's interesting how many children will do that when they feel comfortable about it.

If children complain that they're itchy, and the mom can't find evidence of lice, would you recommend that they use the oil anyway?

As far as I can tell, olive oil won't ever hurt you. It's possible that a child could be allergic to olives, but that would be quite rare. A parent would probably know about it. I had one family tell me that their daughter was allergic to olives, and could they use different oil? I said yes. If a child were allergic to peanuts you wouldn't tell them to use peanut oil.

It's pretty easy to get rid of an adult louse with olive oil, if you do all the steps: If you leave it on for at least six or eight hours, and you comb carefully with the oil in the hair.

Say it's five o'clock at night, and my child comes to me and says "Mom, my head itches, would you take a look?" So, I take a look, but I don't see anything. I would still do the olive oil that night, comb it out the next morning, and then call someone who might have better vision or more experience the next day. That way, if there were any adult lice, you'll have gotten them off the head, so they won't continue to lay more and more eggs. Sometimes even if it's not lice, the olive oil helps anyway, especially if it's itchy, dry scalp.

Can olive oil be used as a means of prevention?

Olive oil can control the problem at a very early stage, which is the best time to control the infestation—before any babies hatch. It's the babies (nymphs) that are difficult to kill. I don't want any babies hatching at all. Remember, lice lay four to six eggs a day. The eggs don't hatch for a good week, so if you do regular checks, you can catch those first few eggs.

What are the chances of getting lice from the movie theater?

Can you? Yes! Especially when the theater's been packed and it's one children's show after another. But I think the probability of getting it at a movie theater is really low. The probability of getting it at an adult movie is almost none.

Here's how it could happen: A child with a bad case of head lice leans against the seat. A louse wants to get off that crowded head to find a new head. It crawls onto the chair. Then it could crawl onto the next head that sits in the seat. The louse is not going to fall out with a hair that falls out. Lice are usually not hanging onto one little piece of hair. A louse usually has its claws on several hairs. A nit might fall off with the hair. Am I terribly worried about that nit? No.

What are some ways a child can prevent a head-louse infestation?

A lot of children play beauty shop. They spend time dealing with each other's heads. I tell them that it's probably not a great idea to play beauty shop unless they really need to play it. I needed to play it when I was a child. It was a good game. I needed to play that game. So, play beauty shop like beauty shops play. Don't switch brushes from head to head.

The only way to prevent a louse infestation is to catch early cases, and that is actually first the parents' responsibility and second the school's responsibility.

What about trying on hats in stores?
Is it possible to get lice from trying on hats? Yes, it's possible, but I'd say it's not highly likely.

Where do most people go to learn what to do about head lice?
A lot of people go to physicians for advice. We expect they will have all the right answers, but they may not be the best source of advice. Many are taking their information from companies that are duping them into thinking that their chemicals work.

What new chemicals have you seen people try?
I've seen ivermectin used both in pill form and topical lotion. I saw a child four days after using the pill form and she had lice crawling all over her head. She used the pill twice. It didn't seem to work at all.

How about the ivermectin lotion?
Those cases I've seen use the topical ivermectin in lotion form also continued to have live lice. But remember, I'm only going to see the people who still have lice.

What other prescription medications have you seen people try?
I've seen a lot of people use Kwell, which contains lindane. I've seen lice crawling all

over children's heads after using it. Because of resistance, it may or may not work. But why use something which could cause serious side effects?

What about using mayonnaise to smother lice?

I wouldn't recommend things that can spoil easily, like mayonnaise. When you're coating your head with something and leaving it on overnight, that's smothering. It's not because there's some magic chemical formula that needs to be on your head for twelve hours. And if you're going to leave something on your child's head for six to eight hours, be careful what you use. Do you want that in your child's eyes? Do you want it in his mouth? Remember, most people with lice are children, not adults.

What about using Vaseline to smother lice?

I've seen a lot of people use Vaseline. Vaseline is hard to get out of your hair. And, as with any smothering agent, you're going to have to use it repeatedly. So, don't use something that's so difficult to work with. You have to work with clean dry hair to get rid of the nits. Unless you get rid of the Vaseline, it's difficult to see the nits.

Can day care centers use olive oil on a child's head during the day, instead of sending the child home?

Having the school do the olive oil would be very helpful if schools were open enough and able to do that. That's a very fine idea. When the oil is on the head, the lice are slowed down, so they're unlikely to move to another child's head.

What about other alternative treatments?

There are a lot of things being sold in health food stores that haven't been tested adequately. There are a variety of oils that could be dangerous to children. I really want everybody to be open to a variety of ideas, but you have to carefully assess what you're hearing. You don't jump on a bandwagon just because one person said "This worked for me." It may not be safe. Anything that kills bugs chemically should go through rigorous tests so that we don't place children in danger. In a time of panic because chemicals aren't working, people will reach for anything.

They want the quick fix. In a time of panic, parents, schools, nurses, and physicians all have to use a lot more care. Step back and ask, "What's worse, my child having lice or using some chemical that could be harmful?" So, don't use kerosene just because your grandmother used kerosene. Don't use gasoline because the people in Puerto Rico use gasoline. You can get rid of lice without endangering or harming your child.

What about tea tree oil?

I have a problem with health food stores selling tea tree oil and anise oil and a variety of things that are supposedly killing lice on contact. These are not things you would use every day like olive oil.

We know that olive oil is safe on nearly all human beings. I have no problem using other types of oils that are not toxic to us. But if they're claiming to kill the lice, not smother, but kill them in twenty minutes, ten minutes, those things should be tested to see if they're safe for humans, and tested to see if they're effective to kill lice at this moment. When you're using something that is poisonous enough to kill a louse, I think that it should be tested before we use it on our children.

I often hear parents say "I'm using all these natural things because I don't want toxins on my child's head." Things don't have to be synthetic to be toxic. There are plenty of natural toxins.

Certain entomologists have told me that

they wouldn't use tea tree oil because it's dangerous. I've had a couple of people use tea tree oil (not the shampoo) directly on their heads. They felt like their scalp was burning and itching and it was horrible. Nix and Rid can burn people's scalps too. I mean, some treatments that we're being told to use can be irritating to the scalp.

How much of what you do is reassurance?

Most of what I do is to tell people they're not crazy, that they're not to blame. They've done the things they're supposed to do. Most people that call me have gone through this long enough to know how to nit-pick. They haven't been successful, because they haven't gotten rid of all the lice. It's hard to visually see a louse and to get rid of it. Most of what I do is to tell them how to get rid of the lice and to encourage them to do it on their own.

I don't charge anything for teachers. I don't charge anything for a lot of families. I want them to get rid of their problem. And most people can do it themselves.

Any final thoughts?

Head lice mostly affect children, not adults. I want to say "Think about what you're doing and what you're saying." I can understand why the National Pediculosis Association would say "Oil doesn't work." Because, if you don't do oil correctly, it does *not* work. Smothering does not work unless you know how to smother. Our goal is to help children. We have to keep our minds open if we really want to help.

The NPA really should find out more about the olive oil protocol before telling people it doesn't work. Schools need to be responsible about regular head checks and dispensing accurate information. Parents need to stay calm and do the work to get rid of lice and nits on their children. In other words, the agenda for everyone ought to be the well-being of our children.

And the chemical companies should be held accountable for the consequences when they realize their chemicals aren't working but continue to advertise that they're 100 percent effective.

8 Frequently Asked Questions

What is Pediculosis?

Pediculosis is the medical or scientific term for a head-louse infestation. Head lice are tiny insects about the size of a sesame seed or smaller. They are wingless, have six legs, and live only on the human head and neck.

How do you get head lice?

Since head lice do not hop, jump, or fly, they migrate through direct contact with an infested person or their belongings. Poor personal hygiene does not cause an infestation.

Where do head lice come from?

Head lice come from other head lice, just like all other species. They do not spontaneously generate and do not come from dirt

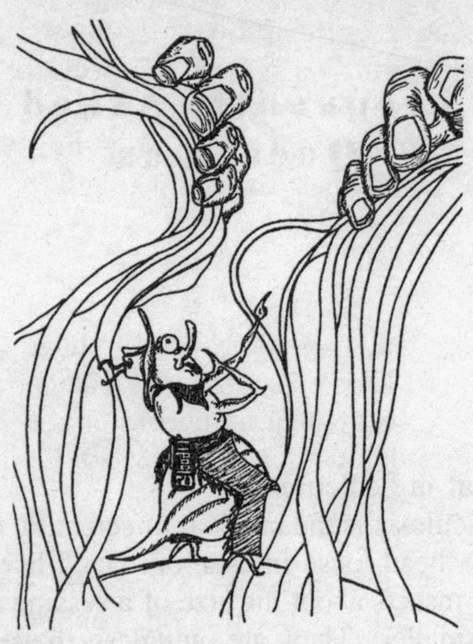

or the air. They have been with humans since prehistoric times.

Can head lice give you AIDS?
No, there is no evidence whatsoever that head lice spread any diseases, including AIDS.

What are the symptoms of head lice?
The most common symptom is persistent itching, particularly around the ears, back of the neck, and crown, but some people never itch at all.

How do you check for head lice?
Use a magnifying glass and check for nits (louse eggs) in bright light. Nits are tiny, almost translucent oval eggs firmly attached to the hair shaft at an angle. Viable nits are usually, but not always, found within a half-inch of the scalp.

How often should I check for head lice?
Check at least once a month, whether your school does regular nit checks or not. Most schools don't have time to do thorough checks on every student.

Do head lice jump from head to head?
No. Human lice cannot hop, jump, or fly.

Can I have head lice if I don't itch?
Yes. Some people are sensitive to the bites, others are not.

How long can lice live off a human head?
About a day but no longer than thirty-six hours. Lice may live slightly longer in hot humid weather than in other climates.

How long can nits live off a human head?
It takes eight to ten days for nits to hatch, but once they hatch, lice need a human

blood meal within forty-five minutes or they will die.

How can I avoid infesting myself when I nit-pick?

When you work on someone's head, it is important to wash your hands and clean under your fingernails before you touch your own head or anyone else's.

Should I heat the olive oil before applying it?

It is not necessary to heat the oil but it is okay to warm it if it is more comfortable. Be sure to test the temperature before applying it to the head.

I used the olive oil and combed out some live lice. Does this mean the olive oil didn't work?

It is not important whether the lice die, only that they are slowed down enough to be caught in the nit comb. The fact that you were able to comb them out means that the olive oil did its job.

I finished the three weeks of olive oil treatments but my head still itches. Does that mean I still have lice?

You probably do not have lice if you followed the protocol carefully, but just to make sure, you should have someone check your head. Your scalp may not stop itching just because you have gotten rid of the lice. The itching is caused by an allergic reaction to the saliva of the lice. It doesn't stop immediately. Also, you may have some other condition and should consult a physician.

Can I get head lice from a swimming pool?
Probably not. When a head louse is deprived of oxygen, it shuts down its system. And when it shuts down its system, it clings to the hair shaft. It does not let go and float to another head.

Can I get head lice from my pet?
No. Pets do not carry head lice. Human head lice do not feed off any species except humans.

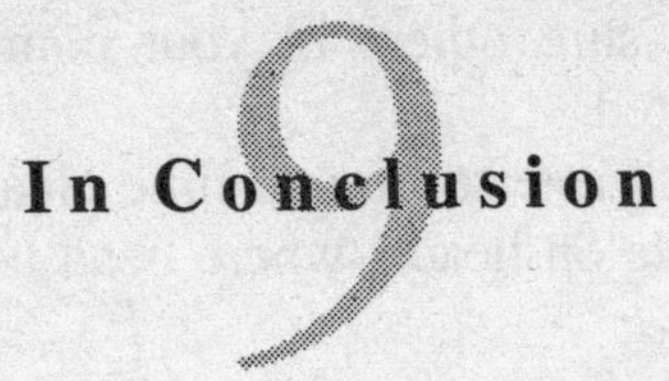

In Conclusion

Head lice are a pain. But they are not dangerous and if you know how to smother them safely, you can get rid of them without making yourself crazy or harming your children. The two best things about head lice are that they are on the outside of the body and they are visible.

The worst thing about a head-lice infestation is that if you don't have enough information, an infestation can make you feel out of control. And an out-of-control parent is not good for the emotional stability of the family.

So, take the time to learn enough about head lice to get back in control, keep your louse-fighting tools handy, and spread the word about the olive oil protocol.

The best ways to deal with head lice are:

- Use simple prevention techniques.
- Catch an infestation early.

- Make sure others in your community are educated.
- Don't waste too much time cleaning. Concentrate on heads, where head lice live and feed.
- When it's over, take a deep breath, pat yourself on the back for another job well done, and get on with your life.

There are other products out there, many advertised on the Internet that purport to kill head lice. We have come across enzymes, sprays, and electric combs that are supposed to zap head lice. Some of these products may be helpful, some are harmful, some are expensive, and others are just plain ridiculous. So, before you invest in any of these products, do your research. Ask questions, and be cautious. In our experience the best investment you can make, besides acquiring knowledge, is a good metal nit comb and a bottle of olive oil.

Consumers need to be very aware that the medical community, the National Pediculosis Association, the American Academy of Pediatrics, and even the media all have their own points of view regarding the treatment of head lice. In the end it is your responsibility as a parent to choose the best treatment program for your family. We hope this book has given you enough background on head lice so that you can tackle an infestation with confidence.

Resources

1) American Head Lice Information Center
215 Lexington Avenue
Cambridge MA 02138
(617) 354-3390
webpage: www.headliceinfo.com
2) Harvard School of Public Health, Laboratory of Public Health Entomology
webpage:
www.hsph.harvard.edu/headlice.html
3) National Pediculosis Association
webpage: www.headlice.org
4) Your local health departments—check your local yellow pages or library
5) 1-888-DIE-LICE
To order the *Head Lice to Dead Lice* book and video, nit combs, or Vision Visors
6) *The Lice-Buster Book*
Lennie Copeland
Warner Books, 1996
7) National Association of School Nurses
P.O. Box 1300
Scarborough, ME 04070-1300
(207)883-2117
(207)883-2683 (fax)

6 June 1997
Joan Sawyer
326 Walden Street
Cambridge, MA 02138

Dear Joan,

I commend your efforts to identify treatments for head lice that are effective, safe, and provide an alternative to traditional methods. As you know, reports from earlier in this century occasionally made reference to olive oil as one component of a more complex formulation for treating infested patients. Olive oil itself has recently been touted by numerous people who attest to its value as one facet in a program designed to eliminate the lice. You convinced us to measure the effect of olive oil on live adult and nymphal head lice. Accordingly, we removed one dozen active lice from the hair of one child, and completely submerged six in olive oil. Lice in oil ceased moving within 5 minutes. Of three lice that were removed from the oil after 1 hour, 2 recovered and regained normal activity. None of the 3 lice treated for 2 hours recovered. The remaining six non-treated lice remained fully active well beyond the duration of this test.

Any insect will undoubtedly succumb to anoxia (lack of oxygen) if submerged in oil for a prolonged period. Olive oil (or other similar product), if applied in copious amounts to the scalp and maintained for a prolonged period, may offer a means of reducing or eliminating the active stages. We have not tested the effect of oil on the eggs (nits).

Your video, "Head Lice to Dead Lice" was informative and amusing. I wish you well in your efforts to identify alternative treatments.

Best wishes,

Richard J. Pollack, Ph.D.
Harvard School of Public Health

The Dead Lice Ditty
T. Sawyer 1997

In order to keep
A louse off your hair
You've got to make sure
That you don't share:

Brushes or combs
Caps and hats
Earphones and ear muffs
Eyeglasses and that's
Not the end of the list.
It goes on—

There's bandannas and beanies
Hairpins and bows
Helmets and headbands
Even sombreros

There's pillows and bonnets
Berets and barrettes
Scrunchies and scarves
Watch out for hairnets!

Make sure that you keep
Your hair off of the rug
Or you'll be a host
To this nit-layin' bug

But if you find them
Don't go into fits

Do eight hours with oil
Then comb out the nits

Work up a lather
Use detergent shampoo
Make sure you don't stop
Till you've scrubbed it all through

Now blow-dry your hair
They can't take the heat
Then search every strand
And in four days repeat

Start with the oil
Then go through each step
Till three weeks have gone by
And you've run out of pep

I've said it before
I'll say it again
The best way to stop them
Is never begin!

EXPERT CHILD-CARE ADVICE AND HELP—

from St. Martin's Paperbacks

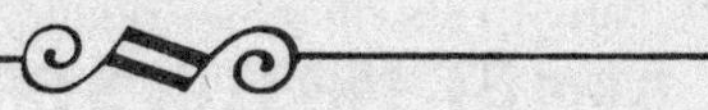

FAMILY RULES
Kenneth Kaye, Ph.D.
Here's how to custom-design a straightforward set of rules on discipline that will fit *your* family.
_______ 95220-1 $6.50 U.S./$8.50 Can.

THE FIRST FIVE YEARS
Virginia E. Pomeranz, M.D., with Dodi Schultz
The classic guide to baby and child care, including answers to the 33 most-asked questions.
_______ 90921-7 $3.99 U.S./$4.99 Can.

BABY SIGNALS
Diane Lynch-Fraser, Ed.D., and Ellenmorris Tiegerman, Ph.D.
There are four distinct styles which infants communicate with—and this book tells you what they are and how to respond.
_______ 92456-9 $3.99 U.S./$4.99 Can.

Publishers Book and Audio Mailing Service
P.O. Box 070059, Staten Island, NY 10307
Please send me the book(s) I have checked above. I am enclosing $_______ (please add $1.50 for the first book, and $.50 for each additional book to cover postage and handling. Send check or money order only—no CODs) or charge my VISA, MASTERCARD, DISCOVER or AMERICAN EXPRESS card.

Card Number____

Expiration date_______________ Signature_______________________

Name____

Address____

City_______________________ State/Zip_________________________

Please allow six weeks for delivery. Prices subject to change without notice. Payment in U.S. funds only. New York residents add applicable sales tax.

CCA 10/97